ABBREVIATIONS COMMONLY USED IN RENAL NURSING

ADH	Antidiuretic hormone
APSGN	Acute poststreptococcal glomerulonephritis
ARF	Acute renal failure
BUN	Blood urea nitrogen
CAPD	Continuous ambulatory peritoneal dialysis
CAVH	Continuous arteriovenous hemofiltration
CCPD	Continuous cycling peritoneal dialysis
CRF	Chronic renal failure
CT	Computed tomography
DN	Diabetic nephropathy
ESRD	End-stage renal disease
ESWL	Extracorporeal shock-wave lithotripsy
GBM	Glomerular basement membrane
GFR	Glomerular filtration rate
GN	Glomerulonephritis
IN	Interstitial nephritis
IPD	Intermittent peritoneal dialysis
IVP	Intravenous pyelogram
IVU	Intravenous urogram
KUB	Kidney-ureter-bladder x-ray
MRI	Magnetic resonance imaging
NS	Nephrotic syndrome; nephrosclerosis
PAH	Paraaminohippuric acid
PD	Peritoneal dialysis
PKD	Polycystic kidney disease
PLN	Pyelonephritis
RPG	Retrograde pyelogram
RT	Renal transplantation
RTA	Renal tubular acidosis
UTI	Urinary tract infection

RENAL DISORDERS

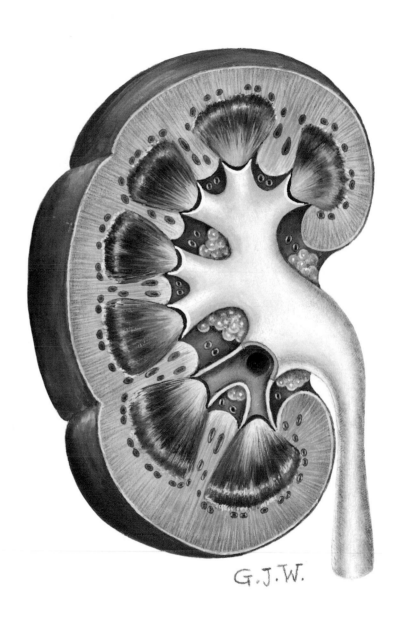

G.J.W.

Mosby's Clinical Nursing Series

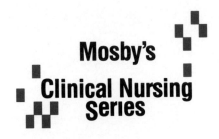

Mosby's Clinical Nursing Series

Cardiovascular Disorders

by Mary Canobbio

Respiratory Disorders

by Susan Wilson and June Thompson

Infectious Diseases

by Deanna Grimes

Orthopedic Disorders

by Leona Mourad

Renal Disorders

by Dorothy J. Brundage

Neurologic Disorders

by Esther Chipps, Norma Clanin, and Victor Campbell

Immunologic Disorders

by Christine Mudge-Grout

Cancer Nursing

by Anne Belcher

Gastrointestinal Disorders

by Dorothy Doughty and Debra Broadwell

Genitourinary Disorders

by Mikel Gray

RENAL DISORDERS

DOROTHY J. BRUNDAGE, RN, PhD, FAAN

Associate Professor
School of Nursing
Duke University
Durham, North Carolina

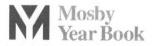 Mosby
Year Book

St. Louis   Baltimore   Boston   Chicago   London   Philadelphia   Sydney   Toronto

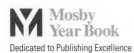

Executive Editor: Don Ladig
Managing Editor: Sally Adkisson
Project Manager: Mark Spann
Designer: Liz Fett
Layout: Doris Hallas

ACKNOWLEDGMENTS

The author wishes to acknowledge the contribution of
Duke University Medical Center to this book . . .
The Department of Pathology: color plates, pages x-xi;
The Division of Radiology, Division of Imaging:
some illustrations in chapters 3 and 5.

Printed in the United States of America

The authors and publisher have made a conscientious effort to ensure
that the drug information and recommended dosages in this book are
accurate and in accord with accepted standards at the time of
publication. However, pharmacology is a rapidly changing science, so
readers are advised to check the package insert provided by the
manufacturer before administering any drug.

Mosby–Year Book, Inc.
11830 Westline Industrial Drive
St. Louis, Missouri 63146

Library of Congress Cataloging in Publication Data

Brundage, Dorothy J.
 Renal disorders / Dorothy J. Brundage.
  p. cm. -- (Mosby's clinical nursing series)
 Includes bibliographical references and index.
 ISBN 0-8016-1685-9

Some data reported here have been supplied by The United
States Renal Data System (USRDS). The interpretation and
reporting of these data are the responsibility of the author and
in no way should be seen as an official policy or interpretation
of the USRDS.

C/CD/VH 9 8 7 6 5 4 3 2

CONTRIBUTORS

Chapter 1, Color Atlas of Renal Anatomy and Physiology,
contributed by

Patricia M. Roberts, B.Sc., M.Sc., Ph.D.
Associate Professor
School of Nursing
Memorial University of Newfoundland
St. John's Newfoundland
Canada

Chapter 3, Diagnostic Procedures, contributed by

Mikel Gray, PhD, PNP, CVR
Clinical Urodynamics
Egelston Hospital for Children
Scottish Rite Children's Medical Center
Shepherd Spinal Center;
Clinical Professor of Nursing
Georgia State University School of Nursing
Atlanta, Georgia

Chapter 13, Renal Drugs, contributed by

Mark Hamelink, MSN, CRNA
Nurse Anesthetist
Morpheus Anesthesia Services, P.C.
South Haven, Michigan

Original illustrations by

George J. Wassilchenko
Tulsa, Oklahoma
and

Donald P. O'Connor
St. Peters, Missouri

Original photography by

Patrick Watson
Poughkeepsie, New York

PREFACE

Renal Disorders is the fifth volume in *Mosby's Clinical Nursing Series*, a new kind of resource for practicing nurses.

The *Series* is the result of the most elaborate market research ever undertaken by Mosby–Year Book, Inc. We first surveyed hundreds of working nurses to determine what kind of resources practicing nurses want in order to meet their advanced information needs. We then approached clinical specialists—proven authors and experts in 10 practice areas, from cardiovascular disease to immunology, and asked them to develop a common format that would meet the needs of nurses in practice, as specified by the survey respondents. This plan was then presented to nine focus groups composed of working nurses over a period of 18 months. The plan was refined between each group, and in the later stages we published a 32-page full-color sample so that detailed changes could be made to improve the physical layout and appearance of the book, section by section and page by page.

The result is a new genre of professional books for nursing professionals.

Renal Disorders begins with an innovative Color Atlas of Renal Anatomy and Physiology. This illustrated review is a collection of highly detailed full-color drawings designed to depict normal structure and function.

Chapter 2 is a pictoral guide to the nurse's assessment of the renal system. Clear, full-color photographs show proper position and technique in sharp detail, aided by concise instructions, rationales, and tips.

Chapter 3 presents the latest in diagnostic tests, again using full-color photographs of equipment, techniques, monitors, and output. A consistent format for each diagnostic procedure gives nurses information about the purpose of the test, indications and contraindications, and the nursing care associated with each test, including patient teaching.

Chapters 4 to 10 present the nursing care of patients experiencing renal failure (acute and chronic), infectious renal diseases, autoimmune disorders, renovascular diseases, metabolic disorders, cancer of the kidney, and obstructive and congenital disorders. Each disorder is presented in a format to meet your advanced practice needs. Information on pathophysiology answers questions nurses often have. A unique box alerting nurses to possible complications provides this information to health professionals in the best position to observe, respond to, and report dangerous changes in patient conditions. Definitive diagnostic tests and the physician's treatment plan are briefly reviewed to promote collaborative care among members of the health care team. Color plates in the front of the book

highlight pathology of selected renal disorders.

Chapter 11 presents surgical and therapeutic procedures, focusing on the nursing care of patients undergoing procedures such as dialysis, surgery, transplantation, and extracorporeal shock-wave lithotripsy.

The heart of the book is the nursing care, presented according to the nursing process. These pages have a color border to make them easy to find and use on the unit. The nursing care is structured to integrate the five steps of the nursing process, centered around appropriate nursing diagnoses accepted by the North American Nursing Diagnosis Association (NANDA). The material can be used to develop individualized care plans quickly and accurately. By facilitating the development of individualized and authoritative care plans, this book can save you time to spend on direct patient care.

In response to requests from scores participating in our research, a distinctive feature of this book is its use in patient teaching. Background information on diseases and medical interventions enables nurses to answer with authority questions patients often ask. The illustrations in the book, particularly those in the Color Atlas and the chapter on Diagnostic Procedures, are specifically designed to support patient teaching. Chapter 12 consists of 12 Patient Teaching Guides that can be copied, distributed to patients and their families, and used for self-care after discharge. Patient teaching sections in each care plan provide nurses with check lists of concepts to teach, promoting this increasingly vital aspect of nursing care.

The book concludes with a concise guide to renal drugs that includes a table of dose adjustments of common drug groups when renal function is reduced. Following is a detailed appendix summarizing nutrition in renal disease. Inside the back cover is a resource section that directs you to organizations and other resources on renal health for nurses and patients.

This book is intended for medical-surgical nurses, who invariably care for patients with acute renal disorders. Critical care nurses in our survey and focus groups also expressed a need for the book. We expect that students will find the book an indispensable help in developing clinical skills and judgment in caring for patients with renal disorders, as it will also be for nurses returning to practice after a hiatus, nurses seeking advanced certification, and nurses transferring to medical-surgical or critical care settings.

We hope this book contributes to the advancement of professional nursing by serving as a first step toward a body of professional literature for nurses to call their own.

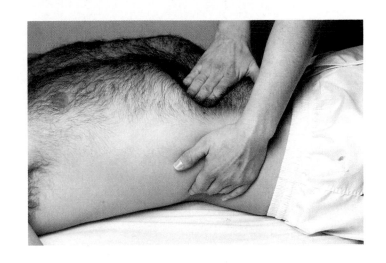

CONTENTS

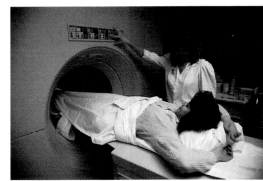

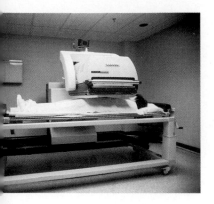

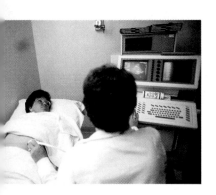

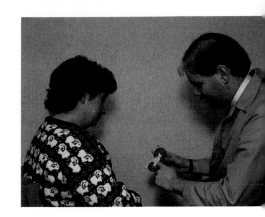

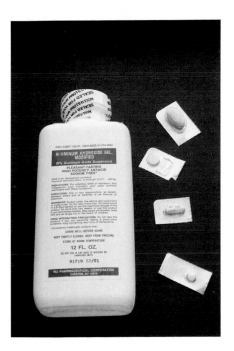

COLOR PLATES

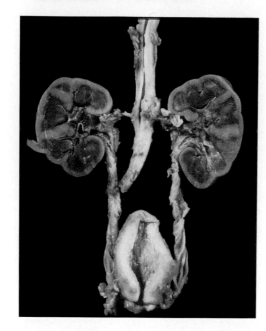

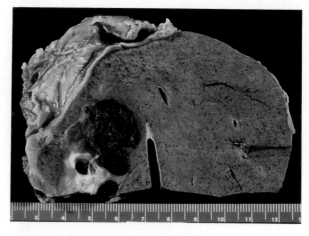

PLATE 2 Renal abscess.

PLATE 1 Normal kidney (also shows aorta, ureters, and bladder).

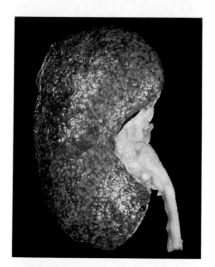

PLATE 4 Malignant nephrosclerosis.

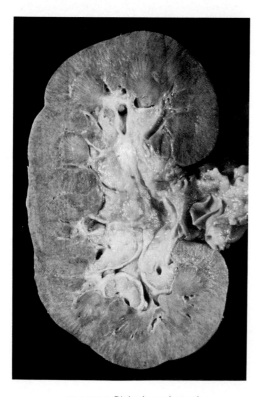

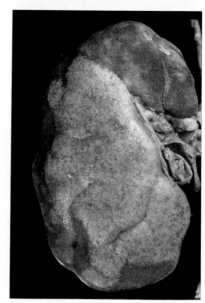

PLATE 5 Renal artery thrombosis.

PLATE 3 Diabetic nephropathy.

Color plates courtesy Department of Pathology,
Duke University Medical Center, Durham, North Carolina.

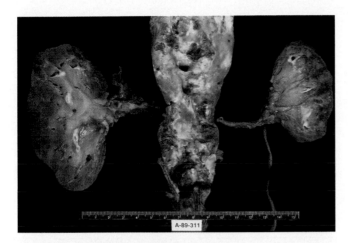

PLATE 6 Renal artery embolism (left kidney)

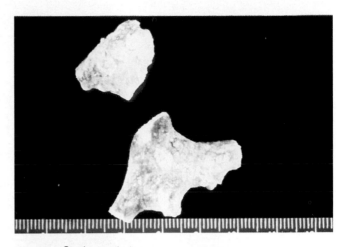

PLATE 7 Staghorn calculus.

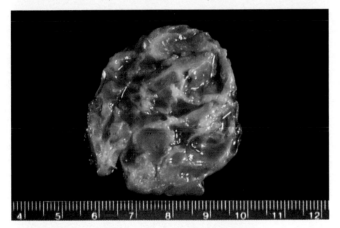

PLATE 8 Renal cell carcinoma.

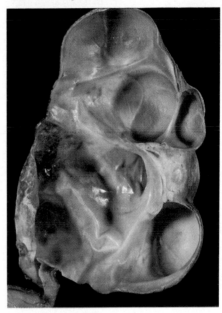

PLATE 9 Hydronephrosis.
Note dilated ureter and pelvis.

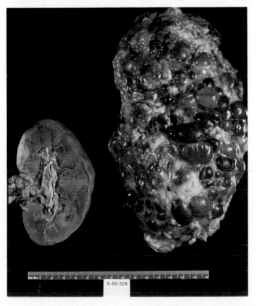

PLATE 10 Polycystic kidney. **Left,** cross section. **Right,** whole kidney showing cysts.

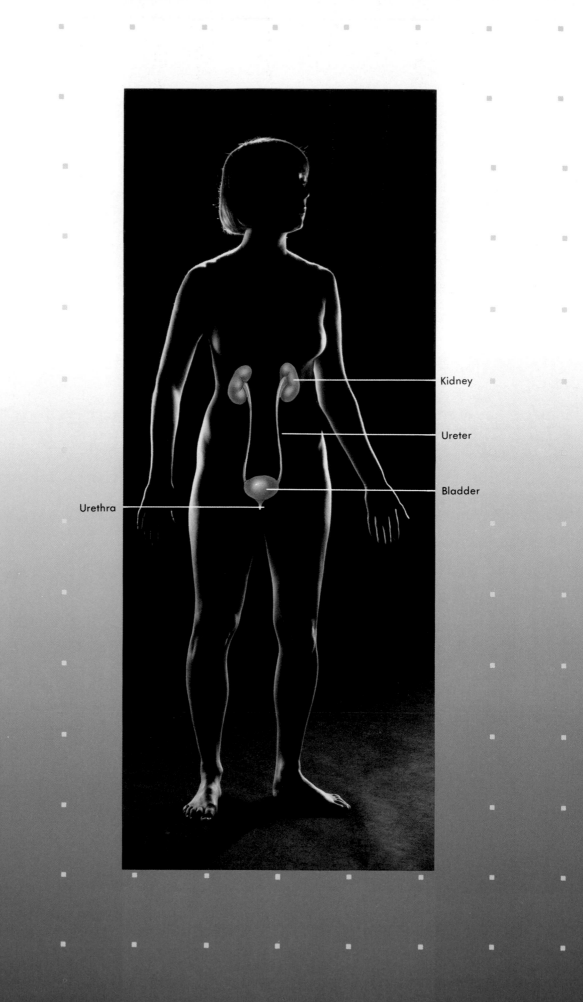

Kidney

Ureter

Bladder

Urethra

CHAPTER 1

Color Atlas of Renal Anatomy and Physiology

The renal system functions to excrete water-soluble waste products and to maintain the homeostasis of plasma water, electrolytes, and pH. Water-soluble blood constituents that can cross capillary walls filter into the nephrons, the functional units of the kidneys, for processing. After this filtrate has passed through the nephrons and collecting ducts, it is called urine. Nephrons process the filtrate by (1) reabsorbing the essential constituents of the plasma filtrate, (2) ignoring the unwanted constituents, and (3) adding other constituents of the plasma to the filtrate by secretion.

The nephrons' ability to maintain homeostasis depends on (1) the circulatory system, which must provide the kidneys with a sufficient volume of blood at the optimum pressure, and (2) the nervous and endocrine systems, which must detect a loss of homeostasis and adjust the intrinsic renal mechanisms appropriately.

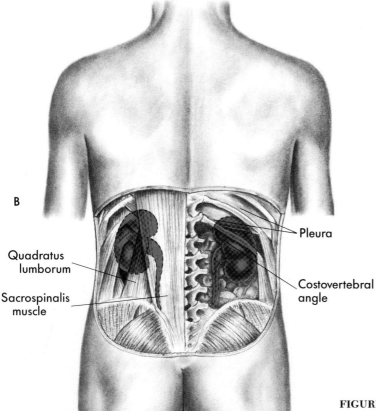

ANATOMY OF THE KIDNEY

The two kidneys are attached by connective tissue and an extensive fat pad to the dorsal wall of the abdominal cavity. They lie outside the parietal layer of the peritoneum, level with the T12 and the L1-L3 vertebrae (Figure 1-1). The renal arteries, veins, nerves, lymph vessels, and ureters all enter or leave the kidney on the medial surface in the indented region called the renal sinus, or hilum (Figure 1-2). (For a picture of a normal kidney, see Color Plate 1, page x.)

The basic structure of the right kidney can be seen in a cross-section in Figure 1-3. The kidneys are enclosed by a strong membrane of white, fibrous connective tissue called the **capsule.** The outer layer of the kidney parenchyma is the **cortex,** which has a granular appearance because of the shape of the many renal corpuscles and convoluted tubules that it contains. The cortex surrounds the **medulla,** which has a fibrous appearance because of the loops of Henle and the collecting ducts of the nephron, which lie parallel to each other in the radial plane. The medulla is organized into **pyramids,** with **columns** of cortical tissue separating them close to the cortex and major and minor **calyces** separating them from the renal **pelvis.** Urine is collected by the pelvis and delivered to the **ureter.**

The **renal arteries** are short and wide to ensure that 20% to 25% of the resting cardiac output (approximately 1,200 ml per minute) passes through the kidneys (Figure 1-4). This is far more than is required to replace the oxygen used by the kidneys, because a larger amount of blood is needed to produce the large volume of filtrate required for homeostasis of the blood. Blood leaves in the renal veins, and lymph leaves in lymph vessels located close to the cortical-medullary junction.

FIGURE 1-1
Anatomic relation of the kidneys to the spinal column. **A,** Anterior view. **B,** Posterior view. (From Thompson.[27])

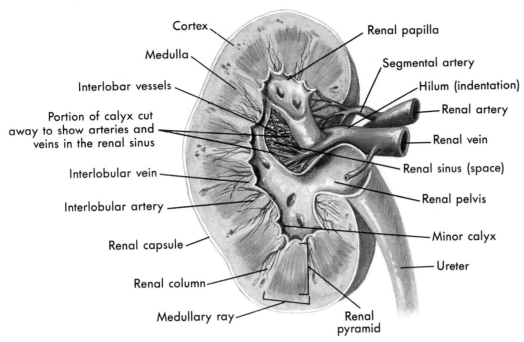

FIGURE 1-2
Longitudinal cross-section of the kidney showing blood supply.
(From Seeley.[22])

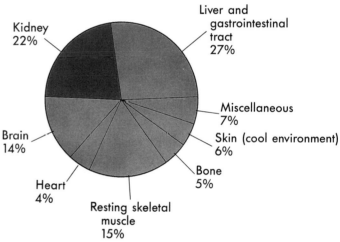

FIGURE 1-4
Proportion of the blood pumped into the aorta
that flows through the kidneys compared with amounts
flowing to other organs of an individual at rest.

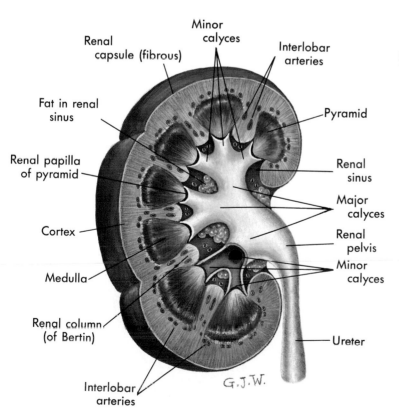

FIGURE 1-3
Cross-section of the kidney showing basic structures.

MICROSCOPIC STRUCTURE OF THE NEPHRONS

The structure of a typical nephron is shown in Figure 1-5. Filtrate flows through the different regions of the nephron in the following sequence: **Bowman's capsule,** the **proximal convoluted tubule,** the **loop of Henle,** and the **distal convoluted tubule.** The nephrons empty into **collecting ducts.** There are two types of nephrons: 20% of the nephrons (**juxtamedullary nephrons**) lie close to the medulla and have long loops of Henle that penetrate deep into the medulla; the remaining 80% (**cortical nephrons**) have short loops of Henle and are located almost entirely in the cortex.

Each nephron has its own **blood supply** (Figure 1-6). Blood is delivered by the **afferent arteriole** to the spherical knot of capillaries that lies in the cup of

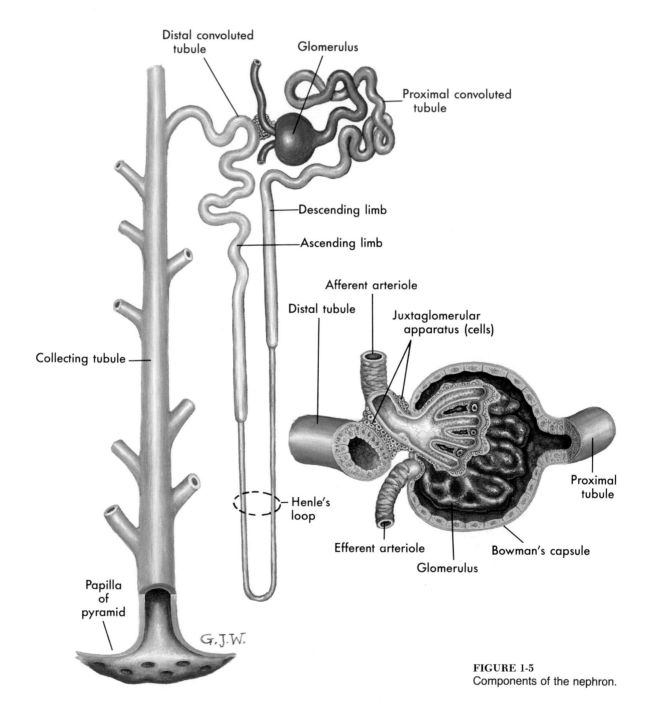

FIGURE 1-5
Components of the nephron.

Bowman's capsule and is called the **glomerulus.** From the glomerulus the blood flows into the **efferent arteriole,** which delivers it to the **peritubular capillaries** that follow the course of the nephron. The peritubular capillaries that loop into the medulla and back to the cortex with the loop of Henle are called the vasa recta. Blood leaves the peritubular capil-

laries in venules that direct the blood back to the general circulatory system.

A patch of the wall of the afferent arteriole is joined to a patch of the wall (macula densa) of the distal convoluted tubule. Together they form a structure called the **juxtaglomerular apparatus,** which monitors and controls the amount of filtrate processed by the nephron (Figure 1-7).

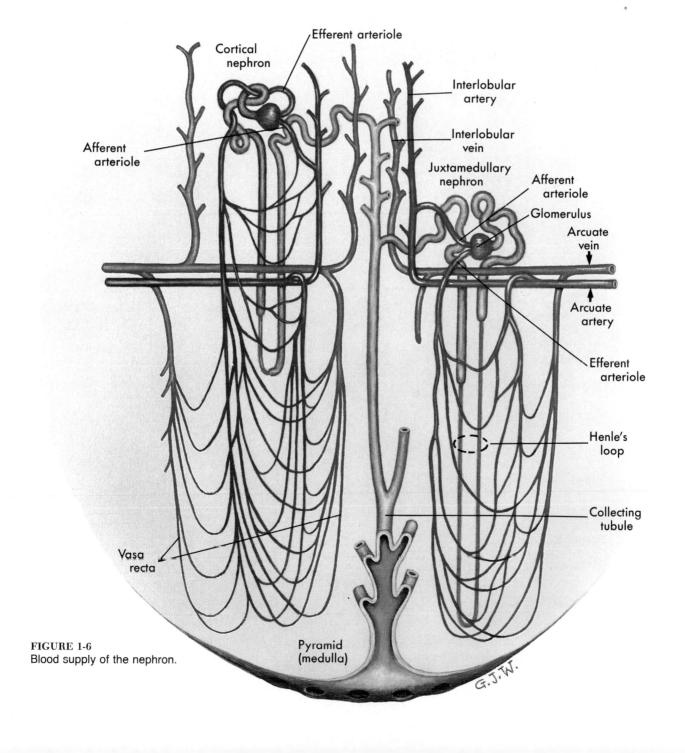

FIGURE 1-6
Blood supply of the nephron.

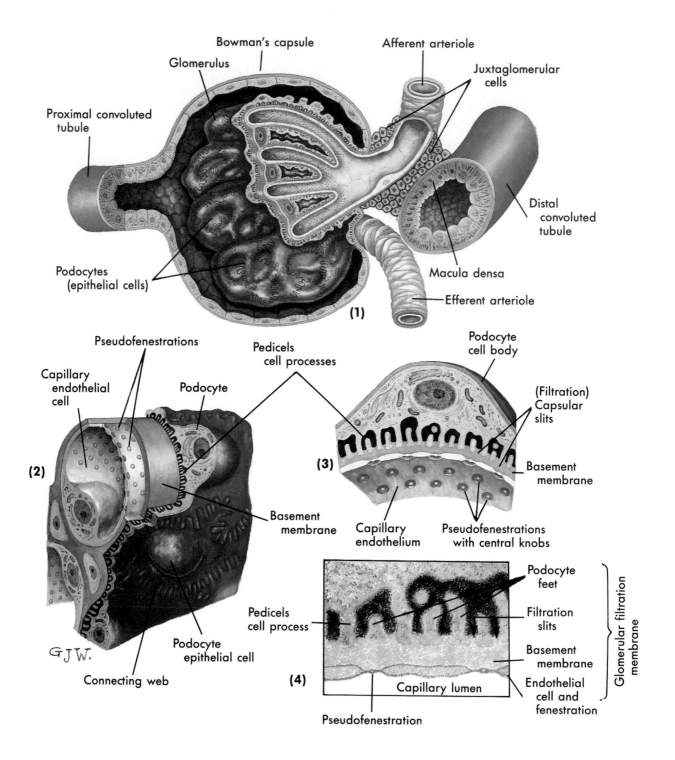

FIGURE 1-7
Renal corpuscle (glomerulus and Bowman's capsule) showing the location of the juxtaglomerular apparatus and the glomerular filtration membrane.

FUNCTIONS OF THE NEPHRONS AND COLLECTING DUCTS

Each region of the nephron is modified to carry out particular tasks. The most important tasks are **filtration, reabsorption,** and **secretion** (see Box). However, the last two processes depend on the first, and homeostasis of the blood can be maintained only if sufficient filtrate is formed. Without filtrate the tubules have nothing to reabsorb and no urine is formed.

The nephrons process approximately 180 liters of filtrate a day and normally can reabsorb all the filtrate's essential constituents because they have a considerable reserve reabsorption capacity. However, there is an upper limit to the quantity of each solute that can be actively reabsorbed. This upper limit is called the **transport maximum,** and it is expressed as the maximum amount that can be completely reabsorbed in 1 minute. For example, the transport maximum of glucose is 225 mg a minute. This is normally reached when the blood glucose rises to 180 mg/dl. At higher concentrations, glucose begins to be lost in the urine.

Filtration is a function of Bowman's capsule, whereas reabsorption and secretion are functions of the tubules and collecting ducts.

BOWMAN'S CAPSULE

Bowman's capsule is shaped like a cup, in which the glomerular capillaries fit snugly (Figure 1-7). The endothelial cells of the glomerular capillaries have large pseudofenestrae (pores), and there are gaps (slits) between the podocytes that form the inner wall of Bowman's capsule (Figure 1-8). These pores and the connective tissue between them form a semipermeable membrane that allows water and small molecules to pass through easily but prevents plasma pro-

---

REGIONS OF THE NEPHRON AND THEIR PRIMARY FUNCTIONS

Bowman's capsule

Filtration: Ultrafiltrate of plasma enters Bowman's capsule and flows into the proximal convoluted tubule

Proximal convoluted tubule

Obligatory reabsorption (approximately 66% of the glomerular filtrate): Sodium, potassium, chloride, bicarbonate, and other electrolytes; glucose; amino acids; water; and urea
Secretion: Hydrogen ions and some unwanted substances (drugs and toxins)

Loop of Henle

Reabsorption (approximately 25% of the glomerular filtrate): Chloride, sodium, and calcium ions; water; and urea

Distal convoluted tubule

Facilitatory reabsorption (approximately 9% of the glomerular filtrate): Sodium, chloride, bicarbonate, water, and urea
Secretion: Hydrogen, potassium, and ammonia

Collecting duct

Facilitatory reabsorption: Water and urea

Note: **Obligatory reabsorption** depends on the maximum capacity of the tubular cells. It is not thought to be affected by hormonal mechanisms. **Facilitatory reabsorption** depends on hormones such as antidiuretic hormone, aldosterone, and atrial natriuretic peptide. **Urea** is absorbed passively wherever its concentration in the lumen increases as water leaves the tubule.

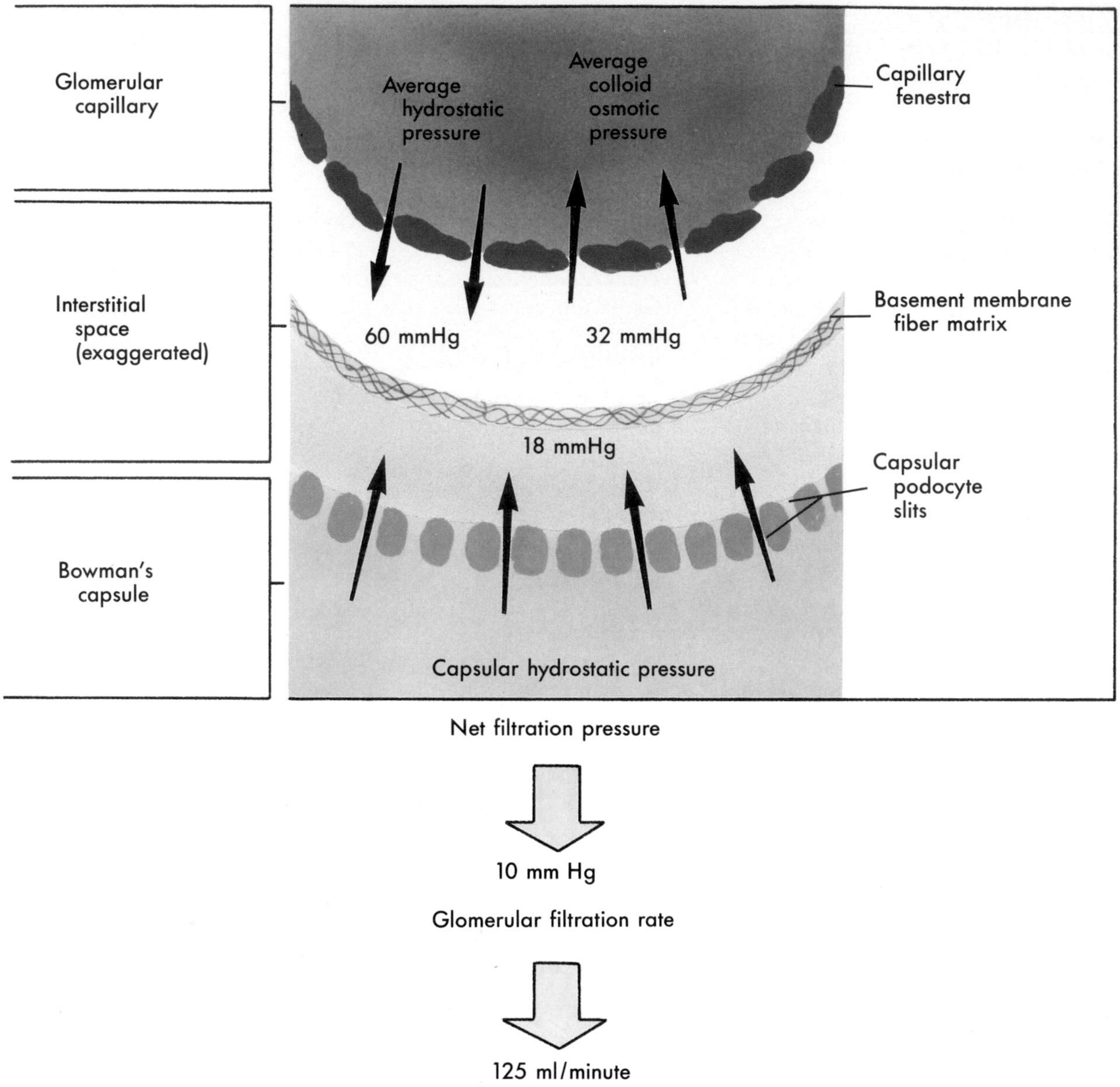

Glomerular capillary

Interstitial space (exaggerated)

Bowman's capsule

Average hydrostatic pressure

Average colloid osmotic pressure

Capillary fenestra

60 mmHg   32 mmHg

Basement membrane fiber matrix

18 mmHg

Capsular podocyte slits

Capsular hydrostatic pressure

Net filtration pressure

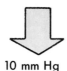

10 mm Hg

Glomerular filtration rate

125 ml/minute

FIGURE 1-8
The three layers of the glomerular filtration membrane, separated to show the pores and the pressures affecting net filtration pressure and thus the glomerular filtration rate.

teins and erythrocytes from doing so. (In some diseases, antigen-antibody complexes are produced that can pass through the pseudofenestrae but not through the capsular slits. These complexes cause an inflammatory reaction that damages the glomerular membrane and allows protein and sometimes even red blood cells to be lost in the urine. If red blood cells are lost, they hemolyze as

they pass through the tubule, and free hemoglobin gives the urine a dark color.)

Approximately 20% of the plasma passing through the glomeruli filters into Bowman's capsule. This is equal to a **glomerular filtration rate** (GFR) of approximately 125 ml per minute (180 liters each day). The volume of filtrate entering Bowman's capsule depends on **net filtration pressure,** which is the difference between the outward push of the hydrostatic pressure and the inward attraction of the colloid osmotic pressure of the blood in the glomerular capillaries.

Hydrostatic blood pressure (capillary blood pressure) pushes against the wall and forces filtrate out of the glomerulus into Bowman's capsule; consequently, the glomerular filtration rate is very dependent on blood pressure. In individuals at rest, hydrostatic pressure in the glomerular capillaries is less than 60 mm Hg, compared with less than 35 mm Hg in other capillaries. Fluid already in the nephron opposes the entry of the filtrate with a hydrostatic pressure of approximately 18 mm Hg. Blood pressure in the afferent arteriole that supplies the glomerulus is so important that whenever pressure falls, pressure receptors in the afferent arteriole activate the renin-angiotensin hormone system of the juxtaglomerular apparatus, which functions to return afferent pressure to its optimum level. Nevertheless, vasoconstriction of the afferent arteriole can reduce net filtration pressure to 0 mm Hg, and activation of the sympathetic nervous system can completely inhibit urine production. This is normal during moderate exercise but can be serious if an individual is under prolonged stress or has a hemorrhage, trauma, or surgery. Therefore it is extremely important to monitor urine production after trauma and surgery, because failure to produce urine indicates that renal function has not returned to normal.

The **colloid osmotic pressure** of blood is approximately 28 mm Hg as it enters the glomerular capillaries. However, if 20% of the plasma filters into Bowman's capsule, the colloid osmotic pressure rises to approximately 36 mm Hg by the time the filtrate leaves in the efferent arteriole. Because colloid osmotic pressure opposes the formation of glomerular filtrate, conditions that reduce it (i.e., by reducing blood albumin concentration) tend to increase the quantity of fluid filtering into the tubule. Blood albumin concentration is kept constant by the

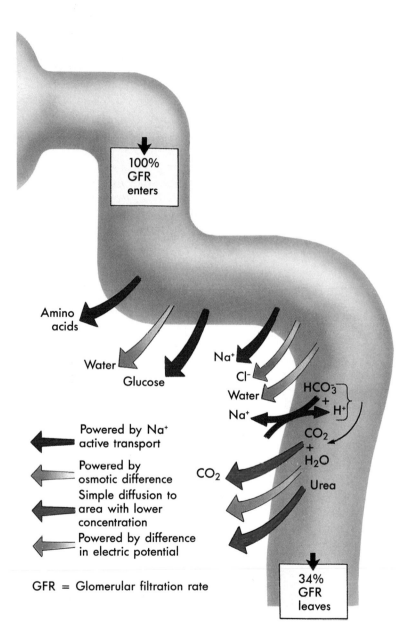

FIGURE 1-9
Active transport in the proximal convoluted tubule.

liver. However, it may fall for short periods when fluid intake is high, or for longer periods when albumin is lost during renal disease or severe starvation.

Net filtration pressure is estimated to be 10 mm Hg by subtracting capsular hydrostatic pressure and glomerular colloid osmotic pressure from glomerular hydrostatic pressure (Figure 1-8):

$$60 - 18 - 32 = 10 \text{ mm Hg}$$

PROXIMAL CONVOLUTED TUBULE

Reabsorption in this part of the nephron is obligatory. The active transport enzymes work at their maximum rate, and the proximal convoluted tubule reabsorbs approximately 66% of the filtrate entering from Bowman's capsule (Figure 1-9). **Sodium** and other cations, **glucose,** and **amino acids** are actively transported out of the lumen of the tubule into the interstitial fluid. **Hydrogen ions** are secreted in exchange for the reabsorbed sodium ions, and they promote the reabsorption of **bicarbonate** because they form carbonic acid, which splits into water, and carbon dioxide, which diffuses out of the nephron. **Chloride** and other anions are pulled out of the lumen by the electrostatic attraction created by the actively transported cations.

Water is drawn out of the lumen by the osmotic pressure gradient created by all the substances transported across the wall of the nephron, especially the large amounts of sodium and glucose, and by the higher colloid osmotic pressure of the blood entering the peritubular capillaries from the efferent arteriole. Throughout the proximal convoluted tubule, the filtrate remains isotonic. Some water-soluble substances, such as **urea,** are reabsorbed because they diffuse passively across the wall after water leaves the lumen and increases their concentration in the filtrate.

If a small amount of protein or other large molecules succeeds in crossing into Bowman's capsule, they are reabsorbed by pinocytosis.

LOOP OF HENLE

Approximately 25% of the glomerular filtrate is reabsorbed by the loop of Henle, although only the ascending limb actively reabsorbs electrolytes, mostly chloride and sodium. The descending limb has a passive role. Because it is very permeable to water and salts, some of the sodium chloride reabsorbed from the ascending limb diffuses across the interstitial space, reenters the descending limb of the loop of Henle, and recycles through the loop of Henle many times (Figure 1-10). The rest of the sodium reabsorbed by the ascending limb enters the peritubular capillaries and veins, along with water that it draws out of the descending limb.

Over time the sodium that recycles in the loop of Henle generates a very high concentration of sodium chloride in the medulla, especially in the tips of the pyramids and their vasa recta, loops of Henle, and interstitial fluid. This high concentration plays an essential role in conserving water during times of dehydration and hemorrhage.

As the hypertonic filtrate moves along the ascending limb from the tip of the loop of Henle, no more water is reabsorbed because the walls of the ascending limb are impermeable to water. The filtrate thus becomes increasingly dilute as sodium chloride is reabsorbed from it. Hypotonic filtrate enters the distal convoluted tubule with an osmotic pressure that is only one third that of the blood and one twelfth that of the tips of the medullary pyramids (see Figure 1-10).

DISTAL CONVOLUTED TUBULE AND COLLECTING DUCTS

Approximately 9% of the glomerular filtrate enters the distal convoluted tubule from the loop of Henle (more than 18 liters a day). It is still too much to lose, and most of it must be reabsorbed to maintain the body's fluid balance. Normally 1% of the glomerular filtrate is lost as urine. Unlike with the obligatory reabsorption in the rest of the nephron, reabsorption in this region is facilitated by intrinsic and extrinsic mechanisms that adjust excretion to maintain the homeostasis of the plasma water, electrolytes, and pH.

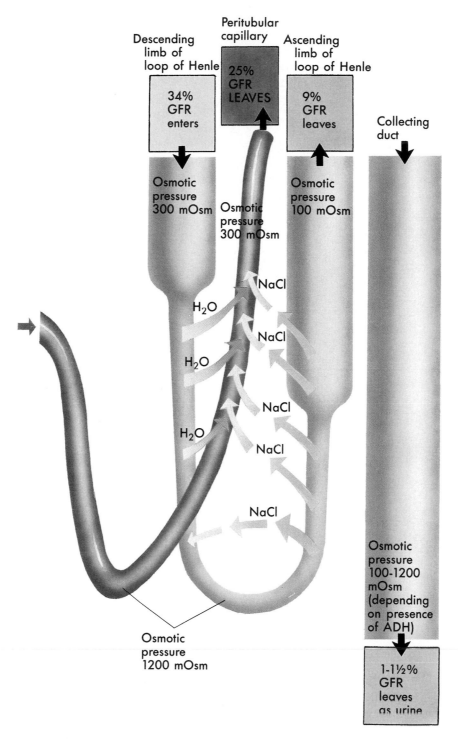

FIGURE 1-10
Diagram showing the movement of water and sodium chloride in the loop of Henle and the osmolalities created.

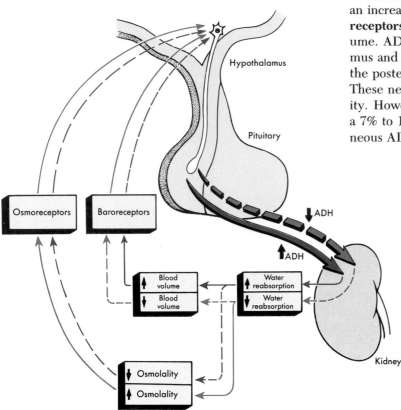

FIGURE 1-11
Relationship between blood osmolality, blood volume, antidiuretic hormone (ADH) secretion, and kidney function. An increase in blood osmolality *(green arrow)* directly affects neurons (osmoreceptors) in the hypothalamus, resulting in release of ADH from the neurohypophysis *(red arrow)*. ADH increases water reabsorption in the kidney, resulting in retention of a greater volume of water in the blood and decreased blood osmolality. Decreased blood volume causes decreased volume in the right atrium; if the decrease is large, it creates a large drop in blood pressure, which is detected by baroreceptors. Nervous pathways (the vagus nerve) carry the information about the drop in blood pressure to the central nervous system and eventually to the hypothalamus of the brain *(green arrow)*. As a consequence, ADH is released from the neurohypophysis. ADH increases water reabsorption by the kidney, resulting in an increase in blood volume. On the other hand, reduced blood osmolality and increased blood volume reduce ADH secretion, resulting in increased blood osmolality and decreased blood volume. (From Seeley.[22])

Homeostasis of Water

Antidiuretic hormone (ADH) is secreted whenever **osmoreceptors** in the hypothalamus are stimulated by an increase in the osmolality of body fluids, or **atrial receptors** are stimulated by a fall in venous blood volume. ADH is produced by neurons in the hypothalamus and secreted from their axons, which terminate in the posterior lobe of the pituitary gland (Figure 1-11). These neurons are inhibited by a decrease in osmolality. However, the ADH secretion that is stimulated by a 7% to 15% fall in blood volume overrides all simultaneous ADH inhibition.

After it is secreted, ADH combines with receptors on the cell membrane of the cells of the distal convoluted tubules and collecting ducts; there, through second-messenger prostaglandins, it increases the ducts' permeability to water. Thus water is reabsorbed by osmosis, because (1) the tubule and ducts contain **hypotonic** filtrate and (2) they pass through **isotonic** regions of the cortex and **hypertonic** regions of the medulla. Thus filtrate and urine are concentrated, interstitial fluid is diluted, and water is conserved. The return of interstitial osmolality and blood volume to their normal set points inhibits further secretion of ADH.

This mechanism is extremely effective and keeps plasma volume and osmolality constant, even though fluid intake varies considerably. Individuals lacking ADH or those whose collecting ducts are insensitive to it (as in **diabetes insipidus**) can produce only dilute urine. Without treatment, they have difficulty drinking enough water to maintain homeostasis of blood volume and pressure, electrolytes, and pH.

Homeostasis of Electrolytes

Electrolytes are compounds that dissociate into electrically charged particles. The major positively charged electrolytes (**cations**) of extracellular fluids (i.e., plasma and interstitial fluid) are **sodium**

and **potassium.** The major negatively charged electrolytes (**anions**) of extracellular fluids are **chloride** and **bicarbonate.** The concentration of these electrolytes in the intracellular fluid is very different from their concentration in extracellular fluid (Figure 1-12). Tissue cells maintain this difference by taking the ions that they require from extracellular fluid and excreting the ions that they do not require into it. Maintaining the homeostasis of these ions in the extracellular fluid is an extremely important function of the kidneys.

The mechanisms that control the homeostasis of sodium are very efficient and can achieve reabsorption of most of the sodium from the filtrate. (Evolutionary pressure created by a shortage of sodium in the diets of our early ancestors encouraged this; now, quite the reverse, North American diets have too much sodium.)

Intrinsic mechanisms include all the local tissue mechanisms that do not require nerve or hormone stimulation to adjust to changes in load. Intrinsic mechanisms that control the reabsorption of sodium are related to the properties of the active transport enzymes (Figure 1-13):

1. Sodium reabsorption in exchange for hydrogen ions increases during acidosis, when plasma hydrogen ions or carbon dioxide concentration increases. This serves to maintain the acid-base concentration of plasma.
2. Sodium reabsorption in exchange for both hydrogen ions and potassium increases whenever excessively large amounts of sodium enter the distal convoluted tubule. Reabsorption of sodium at the expense of potassium does not normally deplete potassium, which is plentiful in a balanced diet. However, diuretics that reduce the obligatory sodium transport enzymes of the proximal tubule and the loop of Henle significantly increase the amount of sodium entering the distal convoluted tubule and may deplete cellular potassium reserves.
3. The juxtaglomerular apparatus plays a role in the autoregulation of its own

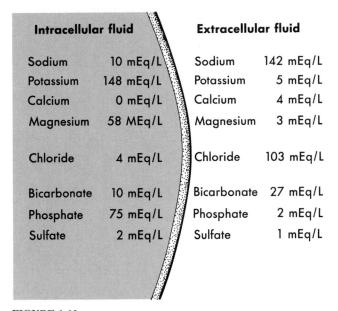

Intracellular fluid		Extracellular fluid	
Sodium	10 mEq/L	Sodium	142 mEq/L
Potassium	148 mEq/L	Potassium	5 mEq/L
Calcium	0 mEq/L	Calcium	4 mEq/L
Magnesium	58 MEq/L	Magnesium	3 mEq/L
Chloride	4 mEq/L	Chloride	103 mEq/L
Bicarbonate	10 mEq/L	Bicarbonate	27 mEq/L
Phosphate	75 mEq/L	Phosphate	2 mEq/L
Sulfate	2 mEq/L	Sulfate	1 mEq/L

FIGURE 1-12
The concentration of some inorganic electrolytes in intracellular and extracellular fluid.

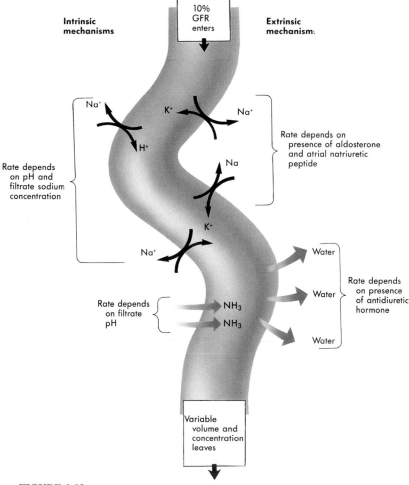

FIGURE 1-13
Intrinsic and extrinsic mechanisms that function in the distal convoluted tubule.

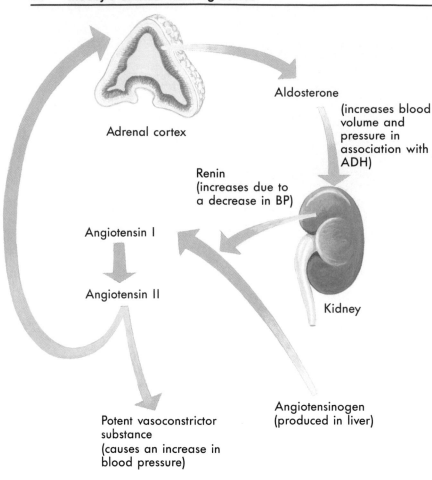

Aldosterone

(increases blood volume and pressure in association with ADH)

Adrenal cortex

Renin
(increases due to
a decrease in BP)

Angiotensin I

Angiotensin II

Kidney

Potent vasoconstrictor
substance
(causes an increase in
blood pressure)

Angiotensinogen
(produced in liver)

FIGURE 1-14
The renin-angiotensin-aldosterone mechanism.

nephron, because it controls the diameter of the afferent arteriole and thus the glomerular filtration rate, so that the quantity of sodium (or chloride) in the distal tubule remains within the optimum range.

Extrinsic mechanisms are mechanisms that involve stimulation or inhibition of the active transport mechanisms by the nervous system or by hormones. These mechanisms are more complex for sodium than for other ions, because the homeostasis of sodium cannot be separated from the homeostasis of water, blood volume, or blood pressure:

1. Much of the osmolality of plasma and interstitial fluid is provided by the sodium that they contain; therefore, because ADH keeps the osmolality of interstitial fluid and plasma constant, it also maintains their sodium concentration.

2. Because ADH alters the amount of water that is reabsorbed, it alters blood volume and pressure, which must also be kept constant.

3. At least two extrinsic renal mechanisms operate to keep blood volume and pressure within the normal range. They do so by controlling the rate at which sodium is reabsorbed by the distal convoluted tubule. If, to maintain the homeostasis of interstitial osmolality (and sodium concentration), inhibition of ADH lowers blood volume and produces hypotension (low blood pressure), the **renin-angiotensin system** increases sodium reabsorption, which then stimulates the release of ADH so that extra water is reabsorbed until blood volume and pressure return to normal. Alternatively, if ADH increases blood volume, **atrial natriuretic peptide** decreases sodium reabsorption, which then inhibits ADH secretion and the reabsorption of water until blood volume and pressure return to normal.

The **renin-angiotensin system** acts to raise blood pressure whenever it falls (Figure 1-14). The enzyme **renin** is secreted by cells of the juxtaglomerular apparatus when they are stimulated by fibers of the sympathetic nervous system or by a fall in afferent arteriole blood pressure. Renin initiates a series of reactions by splitting **angiotensin I** from a plasma globulin precursor, angiotensinogen. Angiotensin I is rapidly converted to **angiotensin II** as it passes through the lungs. Angiotensin II, which is also a potent vasoconstrictor, stimulates cells of the adrenal cortex to produce and secrete **aldosterone.** Finally, aldosterone (a mineralocorticoid hormone) stimulates the sodium-potassium adenosinetriphosphatase (Na/K ATPase) enzymes of the distal convoluted tubule to reabsorb more sodium and secrete more potassium. The extra reabsorbed sodium increases interstitial osmolality and thus increases the secretion of antidiuretic hormone and the reabsorption of water. This in turn increases plasma volume and blood pressure, which exerts a negative feedback on further renin secretion.

Atrial natriuretic peptide acts to reduce blood pressure. It is secreted by cells of the atrial wall when they are stretched by an increase in venous volume. It reduces the reabsorption of sodium by the kidney tubules (Figure 1-15), and consequently extra sodium is excreted. This decreases the osmolality of the interstitial fluid and reduces the secretion of ADH, so that extra water is also lost and blood volume is reduced. This in turn reduces venous volume and lowers cardiac output and arterial blood pressure. It also reduces the tension in the atrial wall and exerts a negative feedback on continued secretion of atrial natriuretic peptide. (This is an oversimplified account of the actions of ADH, the renin-angiotensin system, and atrial natriuretic peptide, all of which have a number of other related effects and are the focus of much current research.)

The homeostasis of **potassium** is also extremely important, because although its concentration in interstitial fluid is low, it has potent effects on nerve and muscle activity. Most of the body's potassium is found within cells, and since more potassium is usually consumed in the diet than is required, the surplus is excreted in exchange for sodium in the distal convoluted tubule. If this is not sufficient and plasma potassium rises, a very slight increase stimulates the adrenal cortical cells directly to secrete aldosterone, which increases potassium secretion into the tubule.

Chloride ions are reabsorbed by the kidneys in two ways: chloride ions are drawn across the wall of the proximal convoluted tubule by the electropositive attraction of the actively transported cations, particularly the sodium ions; and some chloride is actively reabsorbed from the loop of Henle.

Bicarbonate is reabsorbed throughout the kidney tubules as a result of the secretion of hydrogen ions in exchange for sodium. The secreted hydrogen ions combine with bicarbonate in the filtrate to produce carbon dioxide, which then diffuses rapidly into the interstitial fluid. Here the reaction is reversed to produce

Increased blood volume increases atrial wall tension

Atrial natriuretic peptide (decreases sodium reabsorption)

Reduces blood volume and pressure and secretion of ADH

Increases loss of sodium

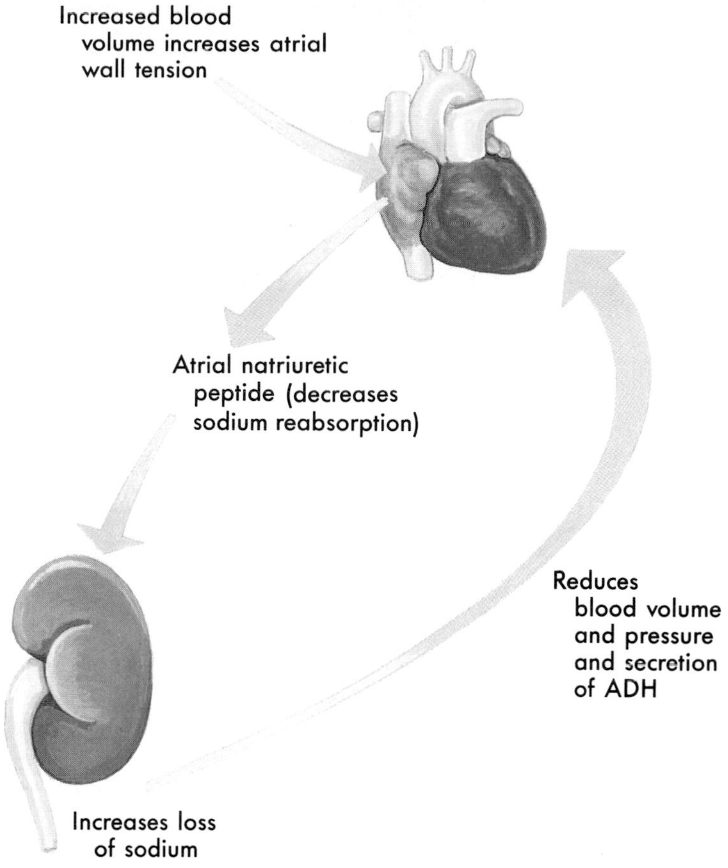

FIGURE 1-15
The atrial natriuretic peptide mechanism.

both bicarbonate to neutralize the reabsorbed sodium and more hydrogen ions for secretion. This reaction is speeded up by the enzyme carbonic anhydrase, which a number of diuretics inhibit to produce their effect.

Caution should be taken in interpreting the results of blood tests that measure the concentration of substances not found predominantly in the blood (e.g., potassium, found predominantly in the cells, or calcium, found predominantly in the skeleton). The amount of potassium in the cells may be below normal, and bones may have lost significant amounts of calcium, yet the blood concentrations of potassium and calcium will be in the normal range because of extremely efficient homeostatic mechanisms.

HOMEOSTASIS OF BLOOD pH

Acids are substances that dissociate to produce hydrogen ions. However, the enzymes of the body are very sensitive to hydrogen ion concentration, which therefore is kept constant by many buffer systems inside and outside the cells. These buffers combine with surplus hydrogen ions or pass them on to another buffer.

Carbonic acid and sodium bicarbonate form the most important buffer for neutralizing strong acids in plasma and interstitial fluid. This buffer is in equilibrium with all the other body buffers, and it is especially useful because the concentration of carbonic acid can be rapidly controlled by the respiratory system, and the concentration of sodium bicarbonate can be controlled by the kidneys. The **normal pH** (hydrogen ion concentration) of plasma and interstitial fluid is maintained by keeping the **ratio** of the concentration of sodium bicarbonate to carbon dioxide at 20:1. This is true regardless of the absolute amount of sodium bicarbonate in the plasma. The total amount of sodium bicarbonate in the blood may vary with different diseases, but as long as the **respiratory system** maintains the **20:1 ratio** by adjusting the concentration of carbonic acid, the pH of the plasma and thus of the other body buffers will be in the normal range. Similarly, the concentration of carbonic acid may change as a result of respiratory disease, but as long as the **kidneys** maintain the **20:1 ratio** by adjusting the plasma concentration of sodium bicarbonate, the pH of the plasma will be in the normal range: **pH 7.35** in venous blood because of carbon dioxide produced by metabolism, and **pH 7.45** in arterial blood because this carbon dioxide was eliminated as the blood passed through the lungs.

The **homeostasis of plasma pH** involves three steps, which are presented in Figure 1-16.

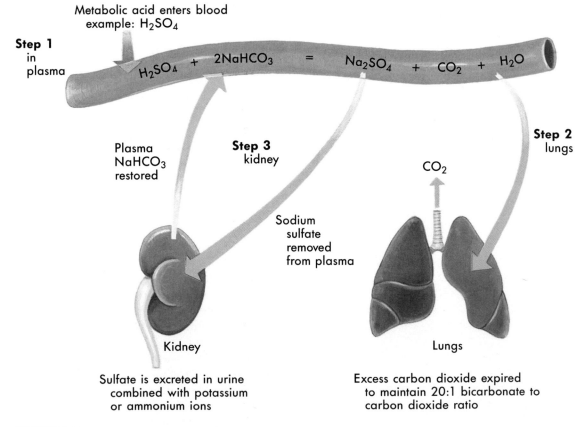

Metabolic acid enters blood example: H_2SO_4

Step 1 in plasma

$$H_2SO_4 + 2NaHCO_3 = Na_2SO_4 + CO_2 + H_2O$$

Plasma $NaHCO_3$ restored

Step 3 kidney

Sodium sulfate removed from plasma

Kidney

Sulfate is excreted in urine combined with potassium or ammonium ions

Step 2 lungs

CO_2

Lungs

Excess carbon dioxide expired to maintain 20:1 bicarbonate to carbon dioxide ratio

FIGURE 1-16
The three processes that maintain plasma pH (hydrogen ion concentration).

Step 1: Strong acids (HA) that enter the plasma and interstitial fluid are neutralized by sodium bicarbonate ($NaHCO_3$) to produce carbonic acid (H_2CO_3) and the sodium salt of the strong acid (NaA)

$$HA + NaHCO_3 = H_2CO_3 + NaA$$

This reaction converts the dissociated and highly damaging strong acid to the weaker carbonic acid, so that the change in the number of free hydrogen ions (pH) is insignificant. However, it does increase the concentration of carbonic acid and reduce the concentration of sodium bicarbonate in the plasma, thus slightly upsetting the 20:1 ratio.

Step 2: The carbonic acid produced in step 1 dissociates into water and carbon dioxide, which stimulates the respiratory system to remove it rapidly. Thus the 20:1 ratio of bicarbonate to carbon dioxide is restored immediately.

Step 3: The sodium salt of the strong acid produced in step 1 enters the nephron along with the other electrolytes. Figure 1-17 shows three acid salts entering the distal convoluted tubule; sulfuric acid is the strong metabolic acid that must be excreted. In the distal convoluted tubule, its sodium is actively reabsorbed in exchange for hydrogen ions split from interstitial fluid carbonic acid. In the renal interstitial fluid, reabsorbed sodium combines with the bicarbonate; in the tubule lumen, the secreted hydrogen ions reconstitute the original strong acid, which is promptly neutralized by ammonia that diffuses from the tubule cells as required. Normally most of the blood sodium bicarbonate used to neutralize strong acids is reabsorbed, and the acid is excreted as its potassium and ammonium salts (see Figure 1-17). However, if large amounts of metabolic acid are produced, some sodium will remain attached to the acid and be lost in the urine.

An increase in the concentration of hydrogen ions and acid anions or a decrease in blood sodium bicarbonate concentration is called acidosis; the reverse is called alkalosis. Acidosis and alkalosis

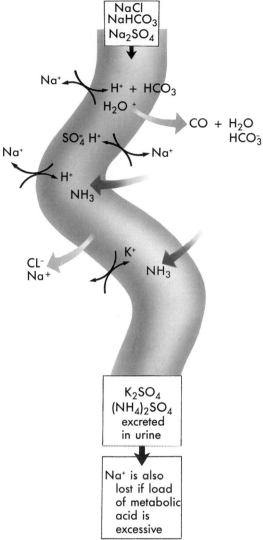

FIGURE 1-17
The handling of chloride, bicarbonate, and unwanted sulfate by the distal convoluted tubule.

are designated according to their cause (Table 1-1). **Metabolic acidosis** refers to acidosis caused by acids produced by metabolic processes (e.g., increased ketoacid production with starvation or diabetes mellitus). **Metabolic alkalosis** may result from ingesting alkali, losing large amounts of chloride during vomiting, or from excessive aldosterone secretion. **Respiratory acidosis** refers to acidosis caused by an increase in the partial pressure of carbon dioxide, such as is produced by impaired respiration or hypoventilation. **Respiratory alkalosis** may be caused by hyperventilation, which decreases the partial pressure of carbon dioxide.

Table 1-1

ACIDOSIS AND ALKALOSIS

Condition	Consequence
ACIDOSIS	
Respiratory acidosis	
Asphyxia	Reduced elimination of carbon dioxide from the body fluids through the respiratory system, resulting in a higher than normal hydrogen ion concentration
Asthma	
Severe emphysema	
Hypoventilation (e.g., impaired respiratory center function caused by trauma, tumor, shock, or heart failure)	
Metabolic acidosis	
Severe diarrhea	Elimination of large amounts of bicarbonate as a result of mucous secretion in the colon
Vomiting of lower intestinal contents	Elimination of large amounts of bicarbonate as a result of production of mucus in the intestine
Ingestion of acidic drugs such as large doses of aspirin	Direct reduction of the body fluid pH
Untreated diabetes mellitus	Production of large amounts of fatty acids and other acidic metabolic end products (e.g., ketone bodies)
Lactic acid buildup (e.g., severe exercise, heart failure, and shock)	Inadequate oxygen delivery to tissue results in anaerobic respiration, increased lactic acid production, and acidosis
ALKALOSIS	
Respiratory alkalosis	
Emotions	Intense hyperventilation as a result of anxiety reduces carbon dioxide levels in the extracellular fluid, resulting in a lower than normal hydrogen ion concentration
High altitude	Decreased atmospheric pressure reduces the amount of oxygen transported in the blood; low blood oxygen stimulates chemoreceptor reflex, causing hyperventilation
Metabolic alkalosis	
Severe vomiting of stomach contents	Elimination of large amounts of acidic stomach contents
Ingestion of alkaline substances such as large amounts of sodium bicarbonate	Raised pH of the body fluids as bicarbonate ions are absorbed
Acidic urine (e.g., drugs such as most diuretics and aldosterone)	Higher than normal loss of hydrogen ions in the urine

(From Seeley.[22])

OTHER RENAL FUNCTIONS

In addition to maintaining the homeostasis of water, electrolytes, and pH, the kidneys are important in the excretion of water-soluble waste products and other substances that the body does not need. A minimum of 25 to 30 grams of urea are formed each day in the liver from the amines removed from amino acids. This urea is excreted by the kidneys, along with other nitrogenous wastes such as uric acid, ammonia, and creatinine. The kidneys also play a role in the transamination and homeostasis of blood amino acids.

Bacterial toxins and water-soluble drugs are excreted by the kidneys, and although most drugs and toxins are inactivated for excretion by the liver, some inactivation is carried out by the kidneys.

The kidneys also serve as endocrine glands. They secrete renin and erythropoietin and play a role in the homeostasis of calcium and bone.

The kidneys produce an enzyme, renal erythropoietic factor, that activates erythropoietin, a glycoprotein formed in the liver and other tissues. This active form of erythropoietin promotes differentiation, proliferation, and maturation of precursors of red blood cells in the bone marrow. Erythropoietin is produced in response to decreases in oxygen tension and renal perfusion that may arise from anemia, hypoxia, or renal ischemia.

Renal prostaglandins are synthesized in the renal cortex and medulla. They appear to be produced in response to both renal ischemia and vasoconstriction. Observations suggest that they participate in the maintenance of renal vascular resistance and the glomerular filtration rate, especially when renal hemodynamics are altered. The complex relationships of renal prostaglandins are not yet clearly understood.

The kidneys also play a role in the metabolism of vitamin D. Vitamin D_3 is formed in the skin, metabolized in the liver to 1-hydroxy D_3, and then metabolized by the kidneys to an active form (1,25-dihydroxy D_3 and others). The 1,25-dihydroxy D_3 is produced in response to hypocalcemia or hypophosphatemia. It acts in conjunction with the parathyroid hormone to increase intestinal absorption of calcium and phosphate, mobilize calcium from bones, and increase renal tubular reabsorption of calcium and phosphate. The production of 1,25-dihydroxy D_3 is suppressed by hypercalcemia and hyperphosphatemia. Production of 1,25-dihydroxy D_3 decreases in chronic renal failure and is considered significant in the development of renal osteodystrophy.

TESTS OF RENAL FUNCTION

URINALYSIS

Analysis of the urine to identify abnormal constituents such as albumin, hemoglobin, visible blood, glucose, and bilirubin provides a simple, noninvasive test of renal function. The presence of some of these constituents (e.g., albumin and hemoglobin) indicates abnormalities in the glomerular membrane; other substances indicate infection or trauma in the urinary tract; glucose and bilirubin indicate diseases originating elsewhere. The specific gravity of urine can be used to determine the kidneys' ability to concentrate urine, and pH is checked to determine whether it is in the normal range. Table 1-2 gives the normal composition of urine.

RENAL CLEARANCE

Renal clearance expresses the theoretical volume of plasma that is completely cleared of the various substances found in urine. For example, although not all the urea is removed from plasma as it passes through the kidneys, the amount normally extracted in 1 minute is equivalent to that contained in approximately 75 ml of plasma; therefore the renal clearance of urea is said to be 75 ml per minute. To calculate renal clearance of a particular substance, its concentration in plasma and the total amount excreted in urine must be measured.

Sometimes compounds are injected into the blood and the renal clearance is calculated to obtain special estimates of

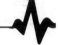

Table 1-2

NORMAL URINE VALUES

Laboratory Test	Normal Adult Values
Calcium (24 hr)	100-250 mg/day (diet dependent; based on average calcium intake of 600-800 mg/24 hr)
Chloride	110-250 mEq/day
Creatinine	Men: 1-2 g/24 hr; women: 0.8-1.8 g/24 hr
Glucose	Up to 100 mg/24 hr
Osmolality	250-900 mOsm/kg
Protein	30-150 mg/24 hr (method dependent)
pH	4.5-8
Phosphorus	0.9-1.3 g/day (diet dependent)
Potassium	26-123 mEq/24 hr (markedly intake dependent)
Sodium	27-287 mEq/24 hr (diet dependent; output is lower at night)
Specific gravity	1.003-1.029 (range in SI units)
Urea nitrogen	6-17 g/day
Uric acid	250-750 mg/day
Volume	Men: 800-2,000 ml/day; women: 800-1,600 ml/day
Color	Pale to darker yellow
Clarity	Clear
Ketones	None
Red blood count	0-5/high-power field
White blood count	0-5/high-power field
Bacteria	None/occasional in voided specimen
Casts	0-4 hyaline casts/low-power field
Crystals	Interpreted by physician
Culture	Negative

(From Thompson.[27])

kidney function. For example, **paraaminohippuric acid** (PAH) provides an estimate of renal plasma flow, because as plasma flows through the kidneys, all its PAH is cleared by filtration and secretion. Renal clearance of **inulin** provides an estimate of the glomerular filtration rate, because the only inulin to be excreted is that which enters the nephron through Bowman's capsule; none is reabsorbed or secreted. Renal clearance of substances such as urea and creatinine can be compared with normal values obtained from healthy individuals and with changes in a patient's glomerular filtration rate to evaluate renal function over the course of an illness.

CHANGES IN RENAL FUNCTION WITH INCREASING AGE

Kidney function is immature at birth. A newborn's kidneys lack the ability to concentrate urine and are less efficient in handling electrolytes. No new nephrons are formed in the kidneys after the fetal period; however, the nephrons and kidneys continue to grow in size until maturity. Thereafter renal weight, blood flow, and glomerular filtration decline, especially after 50 years of age. The changes are most marked when they are standardized to body surface area, less marked when lean body mass is used. As a person ages, the kidneys can maintain the homeostasis of the plasma constituents, but they are slower to respond to changes in load.

When one kidney ceases to function, the remaining kidney is capable of considerable compensatory hypertrophy because there are a large number of reserve nephrons that can enlarge and increase their function. However, the number of reserve nephrons declines with age, and renal parenchyma is replaced by fibrous tissue; consequently, the ability to hypertrophy is reduced in the older individual.

CHAPTER 2

Assessment

Renal nursing assessments require careful, systematic review of the patient's medical, family, social, cultural, psychologic, and occupational history, as well as examination of the urinary system. The interview, conducted in a private setting, allows the nurse to identify the patient's chief complaint, relevant parts of his history, and his response to the situation. The nature of the complaint guides the questioning, and the information obtained should be useful in evaluating symptoms.

This section discusses assessment for upper urinary tract disorders.

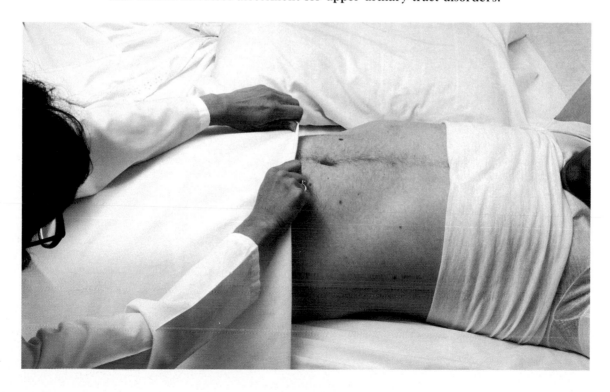

HEALTH HISTORY

CHIEF COMPLAINT: GUIDELINES FOR THE INTERVIEW RELATED TO UPPER URINARY TRACT DISORDERS

Change in usual voiding pattern
  Dysuria: pain or burning on urination
  Frequency of urination: frequent voiding
  Nocturia: need to void at night
  Polyuria: excretion of unusually large amounts of urine
  Oliguria: decreased capacity to form and pass urine
  Anuria: inability to urinate, cessation of urine production
Questions: onset and duration, pattern, severity, associated symptoms, efforts to treat and their
  outcome
Pain
  Location: kidney—flank, costovertebral angle
          ureter—along course of ureter to groin
Questions: character, intensity, onset and duration, precipitating factors, relieving factors, ac-
          companying symptoms
Change in appearance of urine
  Hematuria: bright red bleeding, rusty brown, cola-colored, at beginning, end, or throughout
    voiding
  Proteinuria: deep yellow color, foamy
  Color changes may be caused by food or drugs
Passage of stone
  May be a single stone or gravel-like material; may be associated with hematuria, fever, and
    pain
Patient's perception of problem
  Determine the degree of concern about the symptom, and the patient's opinion as to its
    cause.

Patient history relating to upper urinary tract disorders

Concurrent disorders
Medical history
  Infancy-childhood
  Previous disorders (urinary tract infection, kidney stones, other kidney disease)
  Serious injuries
  Hospitalizations, surgery
  Gynecologic history
  Medications history: current and recent prescription and nonprescription drugs taken
  Family history: polycystic kidney disease, renal calculi, renal tubular acidosis, hypertension,
    diabetes mellitus, renal or bladder cancer
  Diet and nutritional state
  Sociocultural history
  Psychosocial history

PHYSICAL EXAMINATION

ENVIRONMENT AND EQUIPMENT
Stethoscope
A good source of light
Examining table

ABDOMEN

The abdomen contains a number of organs vital to the body. (See Figure 2-5.) The location of the kidneys make them difficult to examine.

Inspection

Have the patient empty his bladder before the examination (both for comfort and to make the examination easier for the nurse). With the patient lying supine, fully uncover the abdomen, leaving the chest covered. Examine the contour between the umbilicus and pubis to detect a distended bladder. Examine the upper right and left quadrants to see if masses are evident.

Auscultation

Using the stethoscope (diaphragm placed lightly on the abdomen), listen in the upper right and left quadrants for bruits over the renal arteries. (See Figure 2-1.)

Percussion

Percuss over the bladder area; dullness over the suprapubic area means urine in the bladder.

Percuss the right and left costovertebral angles to detect any tenderness in the kidneys. Place the palm of your hand over one of the costovertebral angles and strike your hand with the ulnar surface of your fist. (See Figure 2-2.) Repeat on other side. The patient should feel a thud but not experience any discomfort. (This is usually done when examining the back.)

Palpation

Feel for masses and areas of tenderness around the bladder (suprapubic region) and kidneys (right and left upper quadrants), using light and moderate palpation first (Figure 2-3).

Deep palpation is required to feel the outer aspect of an adult's kidney (Figure 2-4). The left kidney may be confused with an enlarged spleen (Figure 2-5). Have the patient take a deep breath. Using the two-hand maneuver, lift the left flank with your left hand and press deeply with the right hand over the patient's left costal margin. The left kidney normally is not palpable. The right kidney usually is easier to feel than the left. For the right kidney, place your left hand under the right flank and have the patient take a deep breath; placing your right hand at the right costal margin, try to feel the lower pole of the kidney. The kidney should feel firm and smooth and should not be tender.

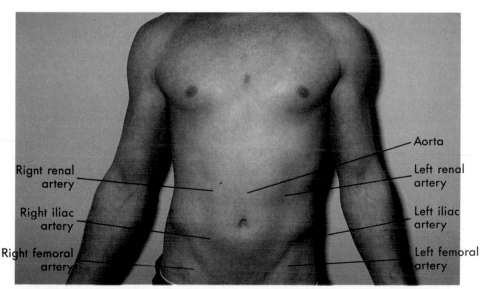

FIGURE 2-1
Sites to ausculate for bruits: renal arteries and aorta. (From Seidel.[23])

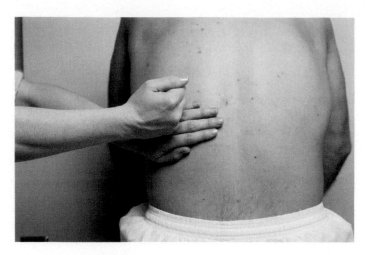

FIGURE 2-2
Percussion of the costovertebral angle.

A

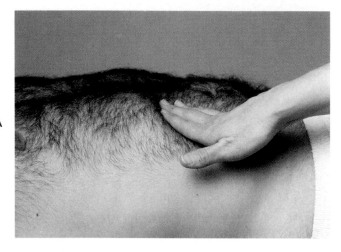

B

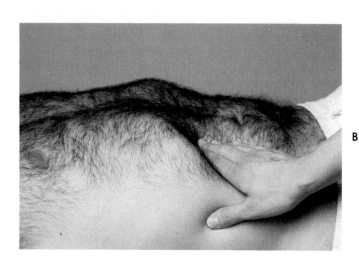

FIGURE 2-3
A, Light palpation. **B,** Moderate palpation.

A

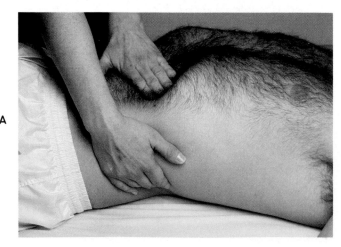

B

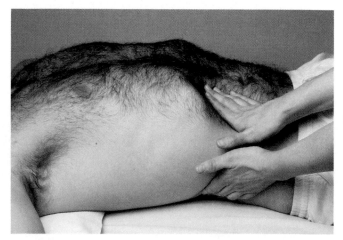

FIGURE 2-4
Deep palpation of the left kidney **(A)** and right kidney **(B).**

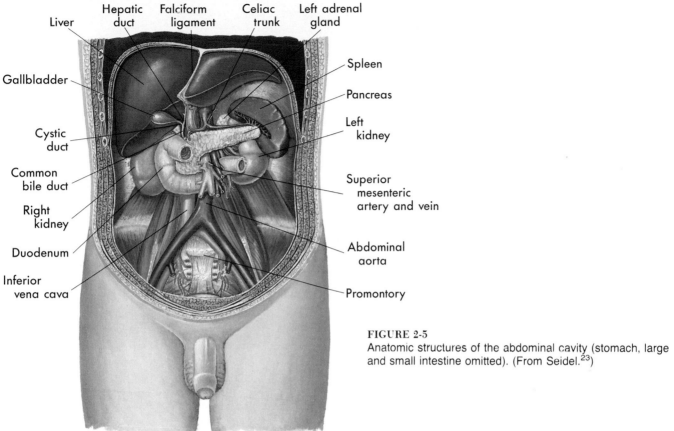

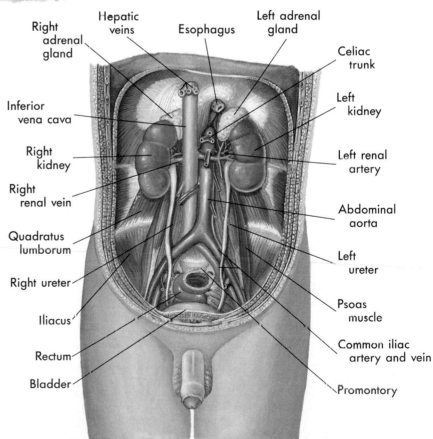

FIGURE 2-5
Anatomic structures of the abdominal cavity (stomach, large and small intestine omitted). (From Seidel.[23])

CHAPTER 3

Diagnostic Procedures

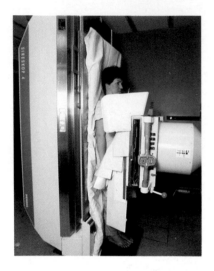

KIDNEY-URETER-BLADDER (KUB) X-RAY

A KUB is an anteroposterior x-ray of the kidneys, ureters, and bony pelvis done without contrast material (Figure 3-1). A single x-ray is obtained from a supine or standing position. A KUB can demonstrate the renal shadows, psoas muscles, pelvic bone, and spinal column (Figure 3-2). It also may reveal radiopaque urinary calculi.

INDICATIONS

Urinary calculi
Preliminary x-ray for intravenous urogram/ pyelogram

CONTRAINDICATIONS

None

NURSING CARE

Preparation for a KUB varies according to the purpose of the study. A "bowel prep" is required when a KUB is done before an intravenous urogram; no preparation is necessary for a KUB done as a single study.

PATIENT TEACHING

Explain the procedure and its purpose, whether as a single examination or as a preliminary x-ray for an intravenous urogram or a voiding cystogram. Describe the procedure, and assure the patient that it is painless and will take only a few minutes. Explain to the patient that the KUB cannot detect radiolucent stones and may not detect small radiopaque ones.

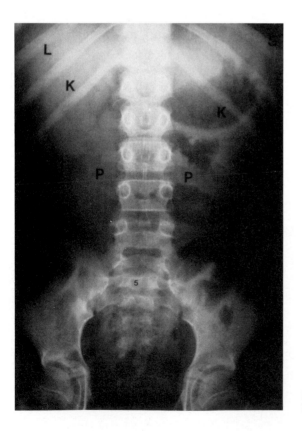

FIGURE 3-2
KUB image. *L,* liver; *K,* kidney; *P,* psoas muscle.

INTRAVENOUS UROGRAM/PYELOGRAM (IVU/IVP) WITH NEPHROTOMOGRAMS

An IVU/IVP is a series of contrast-enhanced radiographic x-rays that provide detailed information about the entire urinary tract, including the kidneys, ureters, and bladder; the kidneys' ability to concentrate and excrete contrast material provides clues to their function (Figures 3-3 and 3-4). Transport of urine from the renal pelvis to the bladder is evaluated by means of sequential x-rays of the abdomen and pelvis taken after contrast material is injected intravenously. (The abdomen may be compressed with a binder to enhance this evaluation.) X-rays of the partly filled bladder provide a limited cystogram; the patient's ability to empty the bladder is evaluated on an x-ray taken after voiding. The IVU/IVP is performed after adequate preparation of the bowel to minimize visual obscurity caused by fecal material and bowel gas in the abdomen. Views obtained during the IVU/IVP are enhanced by using the technique of nephrotomography, which produces a series of x-rays focusing on a single plane of the kidney rather than the nonspecific views obtained by the standard technique. Nephrotomograms are particularly useful for evaluating urinary calculi or renal tumors.

Radiation doses during an IVU/IVP vary significantly, ranging from 1,047 to 1,465 milliroentgens.

INDICATIONS

Urinary calculi
Recurrent urinary tract infection
Febrile urinary tract infection
Hematuria
Renal mass or tumor
Urinary system tumor
Obstruction
Congenital urinary system anomaly

CONTRAINDICATIONS

Allergy to intravenous, iodine-bound contrast material
Allergy to cutaneous iodine-based cleansing solution

CAUTIONS

Diabetes mellitus
Multiple myeloma
Renal insufficiency

NURSING CARE

Patients must be carefully screened for a potential allergy to intravenous contrast materials. If the patient has a history of being allergic to shellfish, consult the radiology department and the patient's physician. Those with potential contraindications for IVU/IVP in-

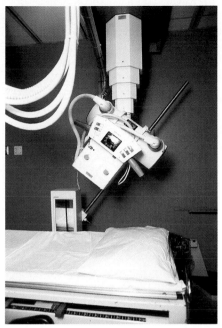

FIGURE 3-3
IVU/IVP equipment.

clude individuals at increased risk for dehydration, either as a result of bowel preparation or because of a disease that predisposes the person to rapid dehydration (e.g., diabetes mellitus, renal insufficiency, or multiple myeloma). The patient's age, health, and patterns of bowel elimination all affect proper preparation for IVU/IVP, which typically involves catharsis and dehydration. **Catharsis** usually is accomplished with an over-the-counter preparation such as Dulcolax or castor oil. In older or sedentary patients, the oral cathartic is combined with a suppository to stimulate more efficient evacuation of the bowel. **Dehydration** is influenced by the patient's age and general health. Elderly patients have fluids restricted for shorter periods of time. Overnight dehydration may be used in adults, and overhydration is avoided.

Individuals with chronic neuropathic constipation may be given a more vigorous preparation. Traditional enemas rely on a bolus of fluid to stimulate bowel evacuation. This technique is less than ideal for IVU/IVP preparation, because it causes gas that further obscures desired views. As an alternative, a mechanical system, such as the Avitar, may be used. It uses a pulsing motion with small volumes of saline warmed approximately to body temperature to produce effective bowel elimination.

After the procedure, carefully monitor the patient for complications, including hypersensitivity reactions and acute renal failure. **Hypersensitivity reactions** vary in severity from transient nausea, urticaria, and itching to respiratory failure and death. Allergic reactions become apparent immediately after the contrast material is injected. To test for this reaction, a small amount of material is injected, and the patient is monitored carefully for urticaria, rhonchi, or shortness of breath. An antihistamine such as diphenhydramine, corticosteroids, and an emergency cart are kept readily available.

Acute renal failure is a rare but serious complication; provide adequate fluid intake, and observe for urinary output of at least 30 ml per hour after the IVU/IVP. Promptly report inability to retain fluids because of nausea and vomiting after an IVU/IVP; dehydration augments the risk of renal failure in susceptible individuals.

PATIENT TEACHING

Explain the procedure and its purpose. Tell the patient that he will be taken to a radiologic suite and placed in a supine position. An intravenous needle will be placed, and contrast material will be injected in a single bolus after a small initial dose to determine immediate allergic response. Serial x-rays will be taken over a period of minutes to hours, depending on the patient's clinical condition and hospital protocols. Warn the patient that he may experience sensations of flushing, an unpleasant taste in the mouth, or nausea as the contrast is given, but reassure him that these responses are transient. Advise the patient that an abdominal binder, producing mild pressure against the abdomen, may be used to enhance the quality of certain images.

If the patient asks specific questions about radiation exposure, advise him to discuss his concerns with the radiologist or attending physician.

RETROGRADE PYELOGRAM (RPG)

An RPG is a series of x-rays that provide detailed anatomic views of the ureter, ureteropelvic junction, renal pelvis, and calyces. The procedure is performed under endoscopic visualization of the ureterovesical junction. A ureteral catheter is placed in the lower ureteral segment, and contrast material is *gently* injected or infused by gravity into the upper urinary tract.

INDICATIONS

Identical to IVU/IVP (RPG is used in patients who are allergic to iodine-bound contrast material or who have nonfunctioning kidneys that are incapable of concentrating and excreting contrast)

CONTRAINDICATIONS

Allergy to cutaneous iodine-based cleansing agents

NURSING CARE

Pyelonephritis related to instrumentation and injection of material into a sterile body compartment is a potentially serious complication of this procedure. Closely

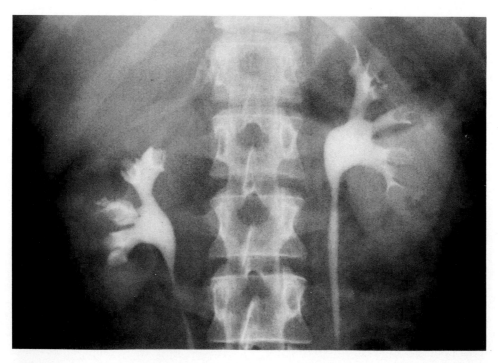

FIGURE 3-4
Intravenous urogram/pyelogram.

observe the patient for flank pain, dysuria, chills, and fever for 24 to 48 hours after the RPG. If symptoms occur, promptly consult the physician and obtain urine for culture and analysis. Administer antiinfective agents as directed. Provide adequate fluid intake after the procedure.

Overdistension of the renal collecting system may produce extravasation of contrast material, causing flank pain and fever. This response typically is transient and disappears within 48 hours, although urinalysis and culture are indicated to rule out infection.

PATIENT TEACHING

Explain the procedure and its purpose. Advise him that injection of the contrast material may produce transient flank pain.

RENAL ARTERIOGRAM

A renal arteriogram is a series of x-rays that allows detailed evaluation of the arterial supply of the kidneys (Figure 3-5). The patient is taken to a radiologic suite, and the skin over the femoral artery is prepared and anesthetized. A radiopaque catheter is threaded through the femoral artery and into the abdominal aorta and renal artery, where contrast material is injected intraarterially. (If passage to the renal artery via the femoral artery proves technically unfeasible, the axillary artery is used as an alternative.) Serial radiographic images over the first 2 to 4 seconds after injection are obtained, providing visualization of the renal arterial system. A nephric phase follows that lasts from 15 to 20 seconds; it is marked by opacification of the contrast material in the renal parenchyma. This in turn is followed by a venous phase, which has limited diagnostic value because of extensive renal extraction and concentration of the contrast material.

Digital subtraction angiography enhances the quality of the study by allowing the use of smaller doses of radiation than in conventional techniques.

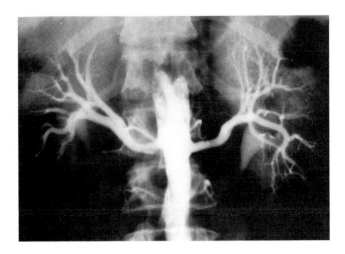

FIGURE 3-5
Renal arteriogram.

INDICATIONS

Renal mass or tumor
Renal trauma
Renal vascular hypertension

CONTRAINDICATIONS

Allergy to intravenous iodine-bound contrast material

NURSING CARE

Preparation before the procedure often includes a narcotic or antianxiety injection to reduce fear. Care after the procedure focuses on preventing complications, including bleeding at the arterial puncture site and allergic reactions to contrast materials. Assess the pedal pulses and capillary filling of nail beds regularly (at least every 1 to 2 hours). The puncture site will be covered with a pressure dressing; assess for signs of frank bleeding until the dressing is removed, 24 to 48 hours after the procedure. The patient is placed on strict bed rest for 4 to 8 hours or more, depending on the physician's judgment and hospital protocol. Advise the patient to expect a hematoma or bruise at the puncture site that will resolve over several weeks. Monitor the patient for hypersensitivity reactions, including shortness of breath and wheezing and rhonchi during and immediately after injection of the contrast material (refer to IVU).

PATIENT TEACHING

Explain the procedure and its purpose, and discuss with the patient any anxiety about the prospect of intraarterial access. Tell the patient that the discomfort caused by intraarterial contrast will be transient. Discuss postprocedural care with the patient, including the need for bed rest and limited movement of the accessed limb during the first 4 to 8 hours after arteriography.

RENAL VENOGRAM

A renal venogram is a set of x-rays of the kidneys' venous drainage system (Figure 3-6). A radiopaque catheter is placed in the right femoral vein and carefully advanced to the opening of the left renal vein. Contrast material is injected, and the catheter is directed upward into the contralateral (right) renal vein and the procedure is repeated. Imaging may be enhanced by injection of epinephrine into the renal artery after venography—approximately 10 seconds later.

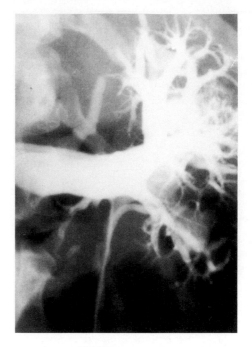

FIGURE 3-6
Renal venogram.

INDICATIONS

Renal vascular hypertension
Renal vein thrombosis
Renal mass or tumor
Congenital anomalies of the urinary system

CONTRAINDICATIONS

Allergy to intravenous iodine-bound contrast material

NURSING CARE

The patient may be given an injection of a narcotic or antianxiety preparation before the procedure. Care after the procedure focuses on preventing or managing complications, including bleeding at the puncture site and allergic responses (refer to renal arteriogram).

PATIENT TEACHING

Explain the procedure and its purpose and discuss with the patient any anxiety about the prospect of intravenous access. Tell the patient that the discomfort caused by intravenous contrast will be transient. Discuss postprocedural care with the patient, including the need for bed rest and limited movement of the accessed limb during the first 4 to 8 hours after venography.

RENAL COMPUTED TOMOGRAPHY (CT SCAN)

A CT scan provides computer-generated axial images of the abdominal contents, including the kidneys, ureters, bladder, and major renal vessels. CT images of the pelvis are useful for detecting and evaluating tumors of the urinary system and enlarged lymph nodes resulting from metastatic invasion. A CT scan provides an estimate of tissue densities, expressed as Hounsfield units; normal parenchyma measures 80 to 100 units. The density of a fluid-filled cyst is lower; solid tumors have a density similar to normal parenchyma. Imaging may be enhanced by injection of a contrast material.

During the procedure, the patient is asked to lie in a supine position while a belt mechanism moves the body precise distances to obtain needed images (Figure 3-7). A single longitudinal view outlines the location of subsequent cuts.

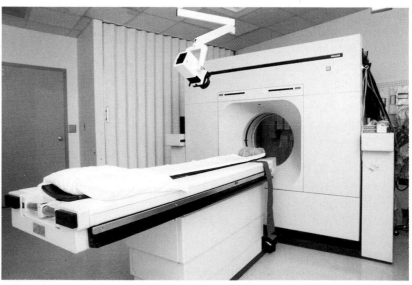

FIGURE 3-7
CT scan equipment.

INDICATIONS

Abdominal mass
Detection and staging of renal tumors

CONTRAINDICATIONS

Allergy to intravenous iodine-bound contrast material
(when injection is needed to enhance imaging)

NURSING CARE

Hypersensitivity reactions may occur when contrast materials are injected. (Refer to Nursing Care under IVU.) Because the patient must remain still during the procedure, sedation is sometimes used for patients unable to cooperate or to understand directions.

PATIENT TEACHING

Explain the procedure and its purpose. Advise the patient that injection of contrast material may be required to obtain needed images. Discuss the need to remain still during the procedure so that serial images are adequately obtained.

MAGNETIC RESONANCE IMAGING (MRI)

MRI consists of computer-generated films that rely on radio waves and alteration of the magnetic field produced by human tissue rather than roentgens for imaging (Figure 3-8). Because of uneven proton counts in living tissues, each tissue creates a small magnetic field. When exposed to a stronger electromagnetic field, the protons align along the field produced by the stronger magnet at the lowest possible energy state. Disturbing the body's normal equilibrium with radio frequency pulses causes a brief rise in the energy state of these protons. When the radio frequency is discontinued, the protons rapidly return to a lower energy state, producing a signal that a computer can detect and thus generate an image. MRI is useful for visualizing the kidneys. Views can be generated from coronal, sagittal, and transaxial planes. MRI has not proven useful for detecting urinary calculi or calcified tumors.

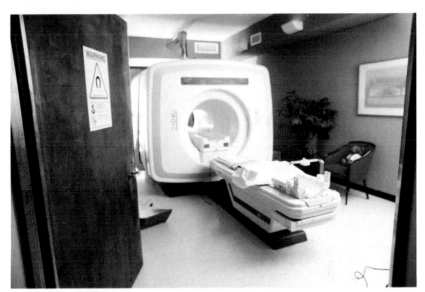

FIGURE 3-8
MRI equipment

INDICATIONS

Abdominal mass
Renal system tumor

CONTRAINDICATIONS

Pacemaker (MRI may interfere with mechanism)
History of aneurysm surgery requiring surgical clips
Other metallic implants (joint replacements) or foreign
bodies (bullets, shrapnel)

NURSING CARE

Preparation for an MRI scan includes a careful explanation that scanning requires lying still in an enclosed tube containing the electromagnet needed for realignment of the magnetic field of body. Consult with the radiologist about sedation of patients with a known history of claustrophobia. Patients who are unable to cooperate or to understand directions may require deeper sedation.

PATIENT TEACHING

Explain the procedure and its purpose. Reassure an anxious patient that the procedure is not painful and that a technologist will talk to the patient throughout the procedure, although the technologist will be unable to remain in the room with the patient. Advise the patient to remove all metal objects that may be drawn into the magnet.

RADIONUCLIDE IMAGING (RENAL SCANS)

Nuclear imaging produces computer images of urinary tract structures through intravenous infusion of a radionuclide tracer substance (Figure 3-9). Renal scans use radionuclide substances injected intravenously that are either bound to renal tubular cells or excreted by glomerular filtration. Renal scans are used to evaluate functional aspects of the urinary system, including the mass of functioning parenchyma, differential function between kidneys, and semiquantitative function of excretory and transport systems.

Following are some of the radionuclide tracers used in nuclear imaging:

1. ^{99m}Tc *DTPA* (technetium-99m diethylenetriamine pentaacetic acid) is principally excreted via glomerular filtration. It is injected in an intravenous bolus followed by sequential, computer-generated images. An initial 30-second image may be taken to determine cortical blood flow. Subsequent images are obtained at 1 minute, and two images are obtained at 5, 10, 15, and 20 minutes, respectively. DTPA will image the kidneys, ureters, and bladder. The scan is used primarily to assess upper urinary tract obstruction, although the glomerular filtration rate, effective renal plasma flow, and differential renal function may be estimated using the DTPA radionuclide. A radionuclide scan provides more functional information than does an IVU but yields less anatomic detail. Imaging of an obstruction is enhanced by injection of a diuretic, such as furosemide, followed by serial images, which allows monitoring of radionuclide washout from each kidney. The computer provides a semiquantitative estimate of washout by producing a graph comparing radionuclide concentration in each kidney over time.

2. ^{99m}Tc *DMSA* (dimercaptosuccinic acid) is bound to the basement membrane of the proximal renal tubule, thus allowing evaluation of the renal cortex. An intravenous bolus of radionuclide is injected, and computer-generated, serial images of the renal parenchyma are obtained.

3. I-131 *OIH* (iodine-131 orthiodohippurate, or hippuran) is excreted in the urine by glomerular filtration (20%) and by tubular excretion (80%). Its use is limited because of the higher doses of radiation (particularly gamma energy) compared with other radionuclides.

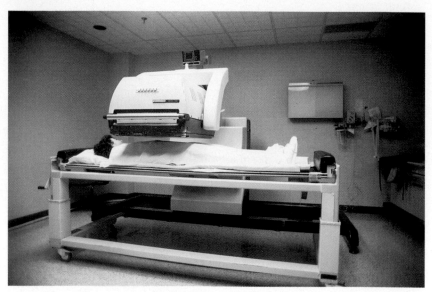

FIGURE 3-9
Renal scan. (From Mourad.[18])

INDICATIONS

DTPA renal scan
Obstruction
Differential renal function

DMSA renal scan
Differential renal function
Detection of renal scars
Hippuran scan
Renal insufficiency

CONTRAINDICATIONS

Pregnancy

NURSING CARE

Radionuclide tracer substances are injected intravenously for renal scans; observe the site for signs of irritation caused by the substance. Bowel preparation is not required. Patients are exposed to significantly less radiation than with an IVU. Nonetheless, since a radionuclide is injected intravenously and excreted via the urine, pregnant women are advised to refrain from caring for patients for the first 24 hours after a radionuclide scan. Consult the radiology department for hospital policies on disposal of urine collecting devices immediately after radionuclide testing.

PATIENT TEACHING

Explain the procedure and its purpose, and advise the patient that the radionuclide scan will provide more detailed functional information about renal function than does an IVU/IVP. Inform the patient of the hospital's policy on disposal of urine collecting devices after a radionuclide scan.

ULTRASONOGRAPHY OF THE KIDNEY

Ultrasonography uses high-frequency sound waves varying from 5,000 to 20,000 hertz (rather than radionuclide counts or x-ray beams) to image urinary system organs, including the kidneys, ureters, and bladder. Ultrasonography offers distinct advantages over radiographic techniques. Since radiation exposure is avoided, a number of images can be obtained, and repeat studies over a brief period of time carry negligible risk. The lack of radiation exposure also means that these tests can be carried out in a physician's office or in a clinic, where lead-shielded rooms may not be available.

Renal Sonogram

Images of the kidneys, renal pelvis, and proximal ureters are obtained from the prone and supine positions. A conducting jelly is placed on the patient's abdomen or back, and axial (transverse) and longitudinal (sagittal) images are obtained (Figure 3-10). The renal sonogram images renal parenchyma, including the pyramids, calyces, and renal pelvis (Figure 3-11). Longitudinal and sagittal measurements of the kidneys can be obtained. Hydronephrosis can be detected, as can dilated ureters, which produce more sonolucent images than do adjacent structures. Calculi are noted when they block transmission of ultrasonic waves, producing a shadow below the area of the stone. Solid tumors are detected when they produce distortion of the renal collecting system and when they contain calcified walls; cysts are noted because of their sonolucent, fluid-filled centers and loculated architecture.

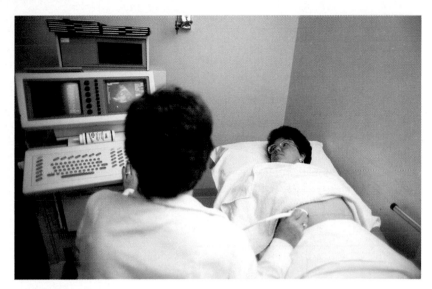

FIGURE 3-10
Ultrasound.

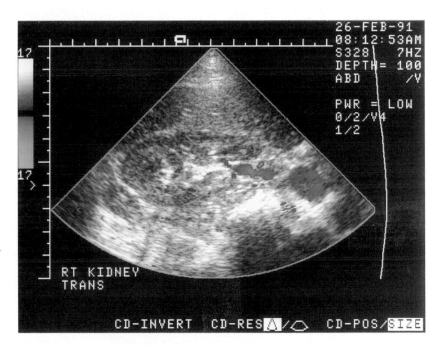

FIGURE 3-11
Image of ultrasound.

INDICATIONS

Abdominal mass
Urinary calculi
Recurrent urinary tract infection
Febrile urinary tract infection

CONTRAINDICATIONS

None

NURSING CARE

Bowel preparation is not required for renal ultrasonography.

PATIENT TEACHING

Explain the procedure and its purpose, and reassure the patient that renal sonograms are painless and noninvasive.

NEPHROSCOPY (RENAL ENDOSCOPY)

Endoscopy is the visualization of hollow viscera in the body by means of light-enhanced telescopic or fiberoptic imaging (Figures 3-12). Nephroscopy allows visualization of the renal pelvis and calyces from an antegrade perspective. A percutaneous tract is obtained before the nephroscope is inserted. In rigid endoscopy, a metal sheath is inserted, followed by introduction of telescopes attached to a powerful light source for visual inspection. Flexible endoscopy uses fiberoptic technology for visualization through a relatively small, flexible, one-piece system. Both flexible and rigid endoscopic

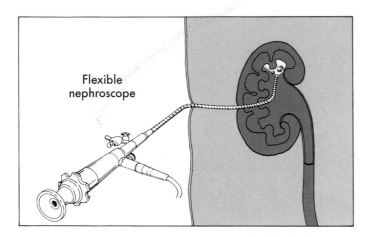

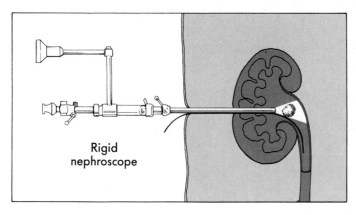

FIGURE 3-12
Nephroscope (rigid and flexible).

instruments provide working ports for obtaining biopsy specimens, for catheterization of ureters, and for other procedures requiring direct visualization of the urinary system. Nephroscopy is often combined with percutaneous nephrolithotomy or ureterolithotomy.

INDICATIONS

Urinary calculi
Recurrent urinary tract infection
Febrile urinary tract infection
Congenital urinary system anomalies

CONTRAINDICATIONS

Current urinary tract infection

NURSING CARE

Careful preparation may include a preanesthesia checklist and assurance of sterile urine. Obtain a urine culture, and treat bacteriuria with sensitivity-guided anti-infective agents under a physician's direction before the procedure. Advise the patient that nephroscopy demands percutaneous access to the renal pelvis, requiring spinal or general anesthesia during dilation.

Complications after endoscopy include bleeding and infection. Assess urinary output after endoscopy for signs of **hematuria.** Immediately report to the physician any evidence of frank bleeding or clots.

Infection may affect only the lower urinary tract or may enter the systemic circulation through minute tears in the urinary mucosa. Assess the patient for signs of systemic infection and potential septic shock, including fever, chills, rapid pulse, and tachypnea followed by hypothermia and decreasing blood pressure during later stages of shock. Immediately report fever and signs of systemic infection before potentially irreversible septic shock occurs. After endoscopy, administer intravenous or oral prophylactic antibiotics as directed. Lower urinary tract infection is noted as persistent dysuria and lower abdominal or back discomfort without fever or chills after the first 24 hours following evaluation.

PATIENT TEACHING

It is essential to explain the procedure carefully to the patient before endoscopy. Consult the physician and anesthesiologist, and explain or reinforce explanations of anesthesia or intravenous sedation that may be used. Advise the patient that he will be placed in a prone position for nephroscopy, which is performed after a tract has been established through the flank.

After the procedure, teach the patient to monitor for signs of urinary tract infection and systemic infection and to contact the physician if symptoms occur.

RENAL BIOPSY

In a renal biopsy a small piece of tissue is obtained via a special needle (percutaneous) or through a surgical incision (open). X-rays of the kidney, ureter, or bladder, intravenous urography, and ultrasonography may be used to locate the kidney for biopsy.

INDICATIONS

Persistent proteinuria
Nephrotic syndrome
Unexplained hematuria
Controlled therapeutic trials of new drugs

CONTRAINDICATIONS

Absolute
Solitary kidney
Irreversible hemorrhagic tendencies
Relative
Uncooperative patient
Suspected renal tumor or cysts
Gross sepsis
Very small kidneys
Horseshoe kidney
Ectopic kidney
Severe hypertension
Massive obesity
Severe spinal deformity
Pregnancy

COMPLICATIONS

Bleeding from biopsy site (i.e., microscopic or gross hematuria, perirenal hematoma, retroperitoneal hematoma, arteriovenous fistula in the kidney, passage of clots, ureteric colic from a clot)
Hypotension
Anemia
Local infection
Pain
Perforation of other nearby structures

NURSING CARE

Record baseline vital signs. Review the chart for hemoglobin and hematocrit levels, platelet count, prothrombin time, and bleeding and clotting times. Review the type and cross-match report for two units of blood. Review the outcome of any test for pregnancy.

Meticulous care and handling of the tissue specimen after biopsy is crucial to the success of the examination.

Consult the pathology department, hospital policy manual, or physician about proper handling of specimens. Label all specimens with the patient's name, the date the specimen was obtained, the source of the specimen, and other information required by the pathology department. Clearly label any specimen obtained from a mass, as opposed to one taken from apparently normal tissue. Give the pathologist a brief clinical history in consultation with the physician.

Measure output carefully and collect the voidings individually. Watch for hematuria. Check for microscopic hematuria, which is invariably present in the first two specimens. The urine may appear pink. Report profuse or persistent hematuria. If no hematuria occurs in the first 24 hours, bathroom privileges can be instituted for the next 24 hours.

A tight dressing is applied to the biopsy site. Check the dressing for bleeding. Apply external pressure for 30 minutes by having the patient lie prone with a sandbag placed directly on the biopsy site. Measure the blood pressure, pulse, and respirations every 15 minutes for 4 hours and then every 4 hours for 24 hours.

Ensure adequate hydration of 1000 to 2000 ml to ensure a good urine flow. Monitor the hematocrit 3 to 6 hours after biopsy. Any decrease from the prebiopsy level suggests perirenal bleeding.

Give a nonaspirin analgesic agent for mild pain after the anesthesia wears off, as ordered by the physician. Report severe loin pain.

PATIENT TEACHING

Before the procedure, prepare the patient for the possibility of pain during the procedure. The patient should cooperate by holding the breath on command. Explain that 24 hours of bed rest is needed after the biopsy, and that some hematuria is normal in the first 24 hours.

Explain the reason for the biopsy and the need for observation after the biopsy. Explain that for several days the patient should avoid contact sports; lifting or heavy exercise; wrestling; riding bicycles, horses, and snowmobiles; and swimming. Normal activities can be resumed gradually after 48 to 72 hours. Explain the need to call the physician if there is any hematuria, draining from the biopsy site, persistent fever, or pain.

BRUSH BIOPSY OF RENAL PELVIS AND CALYCES

A ureteral catheter with a steel guide wire is placed using a cystoscope as a guide. The catheter is then removed, and a steel or nylon brush is inserted to the level of lesion to obtain a biopsy. The specimen is then smeared on slides and prepared with a 95% ethanol solution. After the specimen is obtained, the renal pelvis is irrigated with normal saline.

INDICATIONS

Allows urologist to obtain a tissue biopsy from the renal pelvis or calyces without an open surgical incision to assist in the diagnosis of renal disease

CONTRAINDICATIONS

Current urinary tract infection

COMPLICATIONS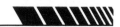

Irritation of the renal system because of manipulation

NURSING CARE

Postprocedural care is similar to that of routine cystoscopic examination. A low-grade fever may be noted. Flank pain secondary to ureteral manipulation is not uncommon and should disappear within 48 hours. Temperatures greater than 38° C (101° F) and severe flank pain should be reported to the physician.

PATIENT TEACHING

Explain the procedure and its purpose. Tell the patient to expect to be placed in a lithotomy position and to have anesthesia. The patient should know how to identify a urinary tract infection after the procedure and to contact the physician should symptoms occur.

CHAPTER 4

Renal Failure

Acute Renal Failure

Acute renal failure (ARF) is a sudden, severe impairment of renal function, causing an acute uremic episode.

Changes in renal function may be considered on a continuum from impairment to failure. Renal impairment may be revealed only by specific urine concentration or dilution tests. Renal insufficiency is revealed when the kidneys cannot meet the extra demands of dietary or metabolic stress. Renal failure occurs when the normal demands of the body cannot be met.

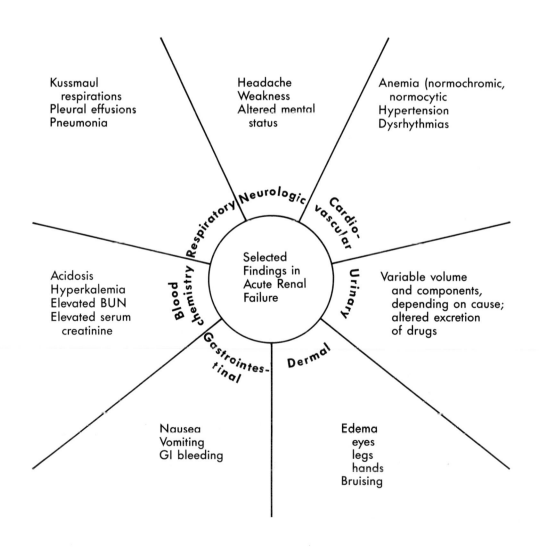

Respiratory
Kussmaul respirations
Pleural effusions
Pneumonia

Neurologic
Headache
Weakness
Altered mental status

Cardio-vascular
Anemia (normochromic, normocytic
Hypertension
Dysrhythmias

Blood chemistry
Acidosis
Hyperkalemia
Elevated BUN
Elevated serum creatinine

Urinary
Variable volume and components, depending on cause; altered excretion of drugs

Gastrointestinal
Nausea
Vomiting
GI bleeding

Dermal
Edema
eyes
legs
hands
Bruising

Selected Findings in Acute Renal Failure

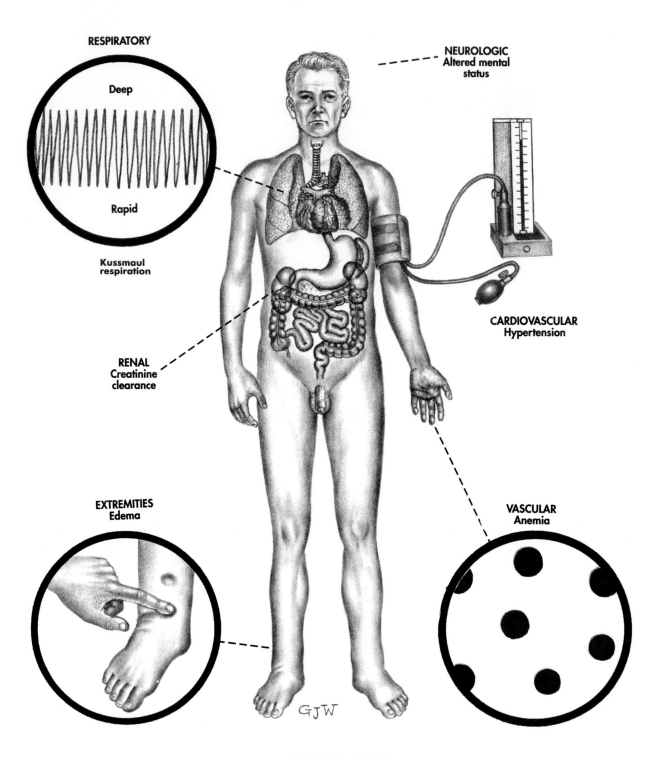

RESPIRATORY

Deep

Rapid

Kussmaul
respiration

NEUROLOGIC
Altered mental
status

CARDIOVASCULAR
Hypertension

RENAL
Creatinine
clearance

EXTREMITIES
Edema

VASCULAR
Anemia

GJW

ACUTE RENAL FAILURE

```
┌─────────────────────────────────────┐
│   NEPHROTOXIC SUBSTANCES            │
│   ASSOCIATED WITH ACUTE            │
│      RENAL FAILURE                 │
└─────────────────────────────────────┘
```

Drugs

Antibiotics
  Aminoglycosides
  Cephalosporins
  Tetracyclines
Antineoplastics
  Cisplatin
  Methotrexate
Anesthetics
  Methoxyflurane
Nonsteroidal
  antiinflammatory
  drugs (NSAID)

Chemicals

Carbon tetrachloride
Ethylene glycol

Pigments

Hemoglobin (hemolysis)
Myoglobin (rhabdomyolsis)

X-ray contrast media

```
┌─────────────────────────────────────┐
│       CAUSES OF ACUTE              │
│       RENAL FAILURE                │
└─────────────────────────────────────┘
```

Prerenal

Hemorrhage
Severe GI losses
Burns
Renal trauma
Volume depletion (actual loss or "third-spacing")
Congestive heart failure, causing decreased renal perfusion
Hypoxia

Intrarenal (renal)

Thrombus
Stenosis
Hypertensive sclerosis
Glomerulonephritis
Pyelonephritis
Acute tubular necrosis
Diabetic sclerosis
Toxic damage

Postrenal

Obstructions (stenosis, calculi)
Prostatic disease
Tumors

(From Thelan.[26])

Health professionals can help detect renal problems early and thus help prevent renal failure. Control of environmental factors such as nephrotoxic substances (drugs, organic solvents, insecticides, and cleaning agents) is important. Safe use and disposal of such agents in industry, agriculture, and the home must be encouraged (see box above). Avoiding unnecessary urinary tract instrumentation could prevent infection. Elimination of predisease factors such as excessive or inadequate urination and fluid intake patterns, urinary tract problems, bacteriuria in pregnant women, and streptococcal infections should be supported. Renal function should be monitored closely in patients with hypertension or diabetes mellitus.

When some of the nephrons are damaged, the normal nephrons remaining are hyperperfused. If this condition goes unchecked, progressive sclerosis of the glomerulus develops, leading to end-stage renal disease. It is believed that restricting dietary protein, if started early, will decrease the hyperperfusion and slow the progression of renal failure. Being alert to prerenal problems in patients with surgery, burns, or trauma helps prevent complications. Genetic counseling may be indicated for families in which a hereditary renal disorder surfaces.

Major causes of ARF include acute tubular necrosis, acute glomerulonephritis, acute urinary tract obstruction, occlusion of the renal artery or vein, acute pyelonephritis, bilateral cortical necrosis, and nephrotoxic agents. A wide variety of substances may be nephrotoxic, including antibiotics (aminoglycosides), anesthetics, iodinated radiographic contrast medium, organic solvents, heavy metals, endogenous toxins, and abnormal concentrations of physiologic substances.

It is helpful to categorize the causes of ARF as prerenal, renal, or postrenal (see box).

Prerenal causes include dehydration, hemorrhage, shock, burns, and trauma; renal causes include glomerulonephritis, acute pyelonephritis, occlusion of the renal artery or vein, bilateral cortical necrosis, nephrotoxic substances, and blood transfusion reactions; postrenal causes involve acute urinary tract obstruction.

Prerenal problems arise from inadequate perfusion of a normal kidney, which can be caused by pump failure, hypovolemia, loss of peripheral resistance, or altered intrarenal hemodynamics. Renal causes stem from primary damage to the kidneys, intrinsic parenchymal damage involving the nephron. Damage can result from acute tubular necrosis, such as that caused by ischemia or toxins; cortical necrosis; infection; major disorders of the blood supply; infiltration (e.g., leukemia); and intravascular coagulation. Postrenal causes involve obstruction of the urinary tract distal to the kidneys, which results in interference with the flow of

PREDISPOSING FACTORS IN ACUTE RENAL FAILURE

Hypotensive episodes

Hypovolemia, renal ischemia from whatever cause

Sepsis, burns, jaundice

Advanced age

Recent surgery (especially cardiac or vascular)

Failure of several organs

Preexisting renal disease or diabetes mellitus

Drug therapy (multiple drugs, aminoglycoside antibiotics, angiotensin-converting enzyme blocking agents)

urine. Such causes may include intrarenal obstruction by crystals, pigments, or Bence Jones protein, or extrarenal obstruction caused by stones or tumors or by hypertrophy of other structures, such as the prostate.

The mortality from ARF is more than 50%.[24] About 1% of hospital admissions are for ARF. Of patients with major trauma or who have had major surgery, 2% to 5% risk developing ARF. The incidence among patients in an intensive care unit is 15% to 35%. Mortality is high despite advances in preventing and treating ARF, and a prime reason for that is the changing population of hospital patients; they tend to be older and generally much sicker.

The prognosis for ARF depends on the cause and extent of renal failure. The mortality rate goes up with sepsis, respiratory failure requiring ventilatory support, and failure of additional organ systems. The very young and very old are particularly at risk. The box above lists predisposing factors that indicate ARF is likely to occur.

ARF frequently occurs in older patients, in whom the typical inciting events are more common. Dehydration is more often a cause of ARF in the elderly or in very young persons than in middle-age adults. Elderly patients with multiple-system problems or preexisting renal insufficiency are particularly at risk.

According to Muehrcke,[19] ARF can be divided into five stages: (1) onset: usually a short time from precipitating event to onset of oliguria or anuria; (2) oliguric-anuric stage: the period during which output is less than 400 ml per 24 hours (usually 8 to 15 days; if longer, the prognosis is poor); (3) early diuretic stage: extends from the time daily output is greater than 400 ml per day to the time that blood urea nitrogen (BUN) stops rising; (4) late diuretic or recovery stage: extends from the first day BUN falls to the day it stabilizes or is in the normal range; and (5) convalescent stage: extends from the day BUN is stable to the day the patient returns to normal activity and urine volume and BUN are normal. This may take several months, and some patients develop chronic renal failure.

PATHOPHYSIOLOGY

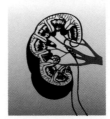

In prerenal azotemia, urinary osmolality is high (greater than 900 mOsm/kg) and urinary sodium concentrations are low (less than 20 mEq/L), which is consistent with renal hypoperfusion and well-preserved tubular function. These findings reflect the physiologic response to hypovolemia or ineffective circulating blood volume. Urinary findings in parenchymal disorders reflect glomerular damage and inability either to conserve sodium (urinary sodium greater than 27 mEq/L) or to concentrate the urine (urine osmolality less than 250 mOsm/kg). In postrenal problems, urinary osmolality and sodium levels may be normal.

Generally, the ratio of blood urea nitrogen to serum creatinine is 10:1. A higher ratio suggests dehydration, gastrointestinal bleeding, increased protein intake, decreased cardiac output, or antianabolic agents.

Damage caused by nephrotoxins appears to affect the proximal tubular epithelium and leave the tubular basement membrane intact. Damage caused by renal ischemia is more widespread and involves patchy areas of epithelial necrosis. Whatever the damage, the glomerular filtration rate (GFR) decreases and urine formation is impaired.

The current explanations for the pathogenesis of ARF include leakage of tubular fluid from damaged tubules into the interstitial areas; tubular obstructions caused by accumulation of intratubular debris or casts; glomerular abnormalities; and changes in renal hemodynamics, primarily excessive vasoconstriction.

Carefully managing fluid volume before, during, and after surgery helps protect renal function; using crystalloid and colloid volume replacement products and blood products helps prevent volume depletion and renal ischemia.

Attempts to maintain renal blood flow (using a low dosage of dopamine) and urine flow rate (through forced diuresis by fluid bolus and diuretics) may prevent hypovolemia from advancing to acute renal failure. The increased urine flow helps prevent casts and other debris from obstructing the tubules. When renal function is at risk, nephrotoxic agents such as the anesthetic methoxyflurane and antibiotics such as the aminoglycosides (gentamicin or tobramycin) should be avoided.

COMPLICATIONS

Hypervolemia	Hypertension
Acidosis	Anemia
Hyperkalemia	Infection
Hyperphosphatemia	

DIAGNOSTIC STUDIES AND FINDINGS

Diagnostic test	Findings
Laboratory tests	
Urinalysis	
pH	Lowered
Osmolality	Hyperosmotic, hyposmotic, or isoosmotic in relation to serum osmolality
Specific gravity	Prerenal: high; renal: low; postrenal: normal
Sodium	Prerenal: low; renal: increased; postrenal: normal
Creatinine	Prerenal: normal; renal: increased; postrenal: normal
Urine sediment	Normal or hematuria; proteinuria; bacteriuria; pyuria; casts
Blood chemistry	
Hemoglobin (Hgb)/hematocrit (Hct)	Anemia; hemoconcentration with dehydration; hemodilution with hypervolemia
Platelets	Decreased adhesiveness
White blood cells (WBC)	Increased with infection
Serum pH	Low-acidotic
Serum bicarbonate	<22 mEq/L
Serum potassium	Hyperkalemia
Serum chloride	Normal or elevated
Serum sodium	Normal or low with hemodilution
Serum calcium	Low
Serum phosphate	High
Blood urea nitrogen (BUN)	Increased
Serum creatinine	Increased
Ratio BUN:serum creatinine	>10:1; prerenal: >20:1; renal: <20:1
Serum osmolality	Increased
Creatinine clearance	Decreased with poor glomerular function
	50-84 ml/min (mild failure)
	10-49 ml/min (moderate failure)
	<10 ml/min (severe failure)
24-hr urine output	Oliguric: <400 ml
	Nonoliguric: 1-2 L
	Diuretic phase: 2-3 L
	Recovery phase: near normal volume
Electrocardiogram (ECG)	Dysrhythmias possible with hyperkalemia or hypokalemia
Kidney-ureter-bladder (KUB) x-ray	Kidney is normal size or slightly enlarged
Renal ultrasound	Kidney size or shape may be abnormal
Intravenous urogram (IVU)	Obstruction, strictures, or masses may be present
Renal scan	May reveal cysts, tumors, or impaired perfusion
Renal biopsy	May be necessary to determine cause and extent of injury

MEDICAL MANAGEMENT

GENERAL MANAGEMENT

The goal of treatment is to try to prevent decreased renal perfusion from progressing to ARF. Fluids and diuretic agents may be used. In any case, the cause of the ARF is determined if possible.

Any reversible components are treated. Failing body systems are supported until recovery. Evaluation for dialysis or transplantation may be necessary if recovery is not complete.

Dialysis, either hemodialysis or peritoneal dialysis, is used to manage fluid volume and electrolyte imbalances (pages 134 to 152); dialysis is particularly necessary with pulmonary edema, hyperkalemia, uremic pericarditis, and convulsions; some nephrotoxic agents are dialyzable.

Hemodialysis is used in hypercatabolic patients to remove nitrogenous wastes and to control serum pH and potassium levels. Peritoneal dialysis is not used in cases involving trauma, infection, immunosuppression, neutropenia, recent abdominal surgery, or severe liver disease.

Continuous arteriovenous hemofiltration is used to remove fluid in an unstable patient, especially an oliguric-anuric patient.

Fluid intake must equal the amount needed to replace measurable losses in urine, nasogastric drainage, wound drainage, and the like; fluid overload must be avoided; daily weights reflect fluid gain or loss.

Packed red blood cells may be needed if symptoms associated with anemia develop; the Hgb level should be higher than 10 g/dl.

Nutritional support should include maintenance of body weight and positive nitrogen balance. A period of negative nitrogen balance cannot be avoided, and weight loss is expected.

Calorie intake should include 100 g of glucose/day. Excess carbohydrate intake can contribute to respiratory acidosis.

Protein intake may be maintained through parenteral infusion of essential amino acids (50-85 g/L solutions); oral intake is started as soon as possible; protein intake is 30-40 g/day with 75% of high biologic value; high-biologic-value proteins are those that contain the essential amino acids in the proportions needed to promote growth, such as milk, eggs, and meat. Serum albumin levels of 3-3.5 g/dl or higher are desirable. Excess protein intake contributes to metabolic acidosis and increased nitrogenous wastes.

Vitamin supplements are needed, since a diet set at 40 g of protein is deficient in calcium and folic acid and low in phosphorus and the B vitamins.

Sodium intake is 500-1,000 mg/day if edema or hypertension is present; potassium in the diet is restricted to 1,500 mg/day if serum levels are over 5 mEq/L.

DRUG THERAPY

Alkalinizing agents: Sodium bicarbonate, sodium citrate and citric acid (Shohl's Solution).

Potassium-lowering agents: Sodium polystyrene sulfonate (Kayexalate), calcium gluconate, sodium bicarbonate, 50% glucose and regular insulin.

Antihypertensives: Clonidine (Catapres), diazoxide (Hyperstat IV), hydralazine (Apresoline), methyldopa (Aldomet), prazosin (Minipress), propranolol (Inderal).

Diuretics: Furosemide (Lasix), hydrochlorothiazide (Hydrodiuril), spironolactone (Aldactone).

Antiinfective agents: Infection is frequently a complication of ARF.
Agents specific to the microorganism cultured should be used.
Agents whose route of excretion is primarily renal should be omitted or used in smaller doses or at lengthened intervals depending on glomerular filtration rate; agents excreted by only the liver require no change; when partial excretion occurs via the kidneys, some adjustment is needed at low glomerular filtration rates.

Phosphate-binding agents: Calcium acetate (PhosLo) and aluminum antacids (which increase gastric pH).

H$_2$ blockers: Cimetidine (Tagamet), ranitidine (Zantac).
NOTE: Particular care is needed in all drug administration (i.e., dosage, interval between doses, and recognition of increased sensitivity) because of altered renal function.

1 ASSESS

ASSESSMENT	OBSERVATIONS
Renal: urine volume in relation to intake	Normal, oliguria, or anuria; change in color, odor
Prerenal problems	Hypotension; flat neck veins, low central venous pressure and pulmonary artery wedge pressure; dry mucous membranes; decreased skin turgor
Renal problems	Hypertension; peripheral edema, jugular venous distention, increased central venous pressure and pulmonary artery wedge pressure; tachycardia
Cardiac	ECG changes related to hyperkalemia: peaked T waves, prolonged PR interval, widened QRS complex, cardiac standstill
Respiratory	Altered rate, rhythm: tachypnea, dyspnea, hyperventilation, Kussmaul respirations; altered breath sounds: rales, rhonchi, crackles; increased sputum production, changes in color; urinelike odor to breath
Gastrointestinal	Nausea; vomiting; anorexia; hematemesis; melena; stomatitis; metallic taste in mouth
Abdomen	Bladder distention with postrenal problems distal to bladder
Hematologic	Pale mucous membranes; pallor
Skin	Bruises; pruritus; dry skin
Neurologic	Change in level of consciousness (somnolence, coma); change in cognitive function; change in behavior; asterixis; seizures
General	Fever; headache; pain in flank or costovertebral angle; muscle cramps; weakness; fatigue; short-term weight changes

2 DIAGNOSE

NURSING DIAGNOSIS	SUBJECTIVE FINDINGS	OBJECTIVE FINDINGS
Altered renal tissue perfusion related to damage to nephrons from hypovolemia, ischemia, toxins, or obstruction	None	Inability to concentrate urine; edema
Fluid volume deficit related to decreased effective circulating blood volume related to active losses and failure of regulatory mechanisms	Complains of weakness, thirst	Hypotension; weight loss; decreased venous filling and skin turgor; dry mucous membranes; tachycardia; hemoconcentration

NURSING DIAGNOSIS	SUBJECTIVE FINDINGS	OBJECTIVE FINDINGS
Fluid volume excess related to sodium and water retention	Describes a change in mental status; dyspnea; anxiety	Hypertension; edema; ascites; anasarca; pleural effusion; abnormal breath sounds (crackles); weight gain; orthopnea; third heart sound; hemodilution; increased central venous pressure and pulmonary artery wedge pressure; jugular venous distention; positive hepatojugular reflex
Altered nutrition: less than body requirements related to gastrointestinal effects of azotemia and restricted dietary intake	Complains of weakness and fatigue; anorexia; nausea, metallic taste in mouth	Vomiting; stomatitis; urinelike odor to breath; documented weight loss
Potential for infection related to suppressed immune response associated with azotemia	None	Signs and symptoms of infection in body excretions, secretions, and exudates; fever; chills; positive cultures of sputum, urine, or blood
Potential for sensory/perceptual alterations; altered thought processes related to endogenous chemical abnormalities associated with azotemia	May describe illusions; may complain of difficulty in thinking, memory loss, and emotional lability; demonstrates apathy or anger	Disorientation to time, place, and person; behavior changes such as altered sleep pattern; altered level of consciousness (somnolence, coma); seizures
Potential for bathing/hygiene and toileting self-care deficit related to side effects of azotemia	Complains of weakness, fatigue	Altered mental status; bed rest ordered by physician
Potential for altered family processes related to health crisis in family member	Talks about inability to adapt to or deal with illness of family member	Family members may avoid visiting or interacting with nurse or physician; may not make use of resources offered such as chaplain, social worker

3 PLAN

Patient goals

1. The patient will demonstrate adequate renal tissue perfusion with a return to a normal or stable level of renal function.
2. The patient will demonstrate a normal fluid balance.
3. The patient will demonstrate adequate nutritional intake.
4. The patient will be free of infection.
5. The patient will demonstrate normal responses to sensory and perceptual stimuli and normal thought processes.
6. The patient will resume activities of daily living without limitations.
7. The patient's family will demonstrate positive adaptation to the family member's illness and recovery.
8. The patient will demonstrate increased knowledge of acute renal failure, its causes, manifestations, and treatment, the need for medical follow-up, and the potential need for dialysis or transplantation in the future.

4 IMPLEMENT

NURSING DIAGNOSIS	NURSING INTERVENTIONS	RATIONALE
Altered renal tissue perfusion related to damage to nephrons from hypovolemia, ischemia, toxins, or obstruction	Assess for Chvostek's or Trousseau's sign; assess respirations.	To identify tetany, hypocalcemia, and Kussmaul respirations (acidosis).
	Monitor laboratory values: serum pH, sodium, potassium, calcium, bicarbonate, chloride, magnesium, BUN, and serum creatinine.	Levels reflect kidneys' ability to excrete nitrogenous wastes, excess fluids, and electrolytes.
	Administer medications as ordered with care; monitor response to drugs.	Dosages of medications may be less than usual, and intervals between doses may be lengthened; monitoring determines the effectiveness of the drug and its dosage and timing and helps identify adverse side effects.
	Avoid nephrotoxic drugs.	Kidneys are less able to excrete drugs they normally eliminate.
Fluid volume deficit related to decreased effective circulating blood volume related to active losses and failure of regulatory mechanisms	Assess neck veins, capillary refill, oral mucous membranes, skin turgor. Monitor weight daily, also 24-h intake and output; assess blood pressure, pulse, and respirations q 6-8 h; assess central venous pressure and pulmonary artery wedge pressure q 6-12 h.	To identify changes in fluid status.
	Monitor laboratory data: serum sodium, potassium, chloride, and bicarbonate.	To identify electrolytes lost through body fluid losses.
	Administer medications as ordered (vasoconstrictors, fluids, and electrolyte replacements).	To increase systemic resistance and blood pressure and thus renal blood flow, and to replace losses and ensure adequate circulating volume.

NURSING DIAGNOSIS	NURSING INTERVENTIONS	RATIONALE
Fluid volume excess related to sodium and water retention	Assess weight daily, also 24-h intake and output; assess blood pressure, pulse, and respirations, including breath sounds, q 6-8 h. Monitor edema, jugular venous distention and, if necessary, central venous pressure and pulmonary artery wedge pressure.	To recognize altered fluid status.
	Monitor laboratory values: serum potassium.	May be lowered by vigorous diuretic therapy.
	Monitor ECG.	Increase or decrease in potassium may be associated with dysrhythmias.
	Administer diuretics as ordered; monitor response.	To determine the effect of drugs and observe for side effects such as hypokalemia and ototoxicity.
Altered nutrition: less than body requirements related to gastrointestinal effects of azotemia and restricted dietary intake	Assess food intake, dry weight.	To assure adequate intake within the limits prescribed; weight is assessed to determine if changes are related to fluid balance or to inadequate caloric intake and loss of muscle mass.
	Monitor for nausea, vomiting, and anorexia.	These conditions increase loss of needed nutrients.
	Monitor laboratory data: serum protein, lipids, potassium, and calcium.	To determine if protein intake is adequate.
	Encourage food intake as prescribed or administer enteral or parenteral feedings; refer complex problems to dietitian.	A team approach to managing the complex renal diet is helpful to all concerned.
	Provide oral hygiene regularly.	To improve taste in mouth.
Potential for infection related to suppressed immune response associated with azotemia	Assess for signs and symptoms of infection in secretions, excretions, and exudates; assess for fever.	To detect any infection early.
	Monitor laboratory data: WBC. Monitor temperature q 4-6 h.	May be increased only slightly in azotemia.
	Wash hands thoroughly and consistently; avoid exposing patient to people with infection; ensure aseptic technique for any invasive procedure or wound care.	To decrease chances for infection.
	Encourage regular oral hygiene, hand washing, bathing, adequate rest, and nutrition.	To help prevent infections.

NURSING DIAGNOSIS	NURSING INTERVENTIONS	RATIONALE
Potential for sensory/perceptual alterations; altered thought processes related to endogenous chemical abnormalities associated with azotemia	Assess orientation to time, place, and person.	This knowledge is lost as mental status is increasingly altered.
	Monitor level of consciousness; observe for changes in behavior; be alert to possible seizures.	Indicates alteration in brain function.
	Orient patient to reality.	To decrease the possibility that disorientation is due to isolation and lack of information.
	Maintain safety precautions: bed rails up, bed lowered, sharp objects out of reach, call bell within reach.	To provide a safe environment and prevent injury.
Potential for bathing/hygiene, toileting self-care deficit related to side effects of azotemia	Assess need for assistance; assist with care as needed.	To help patient return to self-care as appropriate.
	Implement measures such as deep breathing, coughing, and turning.	To prevent adverse side effects of bed rest, such as pneumonia.
Potential for altered family processes related to health crisis in family member	Assess family structure and role relationships; monitor family's response to the illness, treatment, and prognosis.	To identify family strengths and potential problems.
	Encourage verbalization of needs and concerns; discuss impact on roles and adaptation required; identify family strengths; assist with problem solving; support family's decisions.	Crisis intervention may be all that is needed.
	Refer patient and family to other services as appropriate.	To help resolve problems requiring time and skills beyond the nurse's capabilities.
Knowledge deficit	See Patient Teaching.	

5 EVALUATE

PATIENT OUTCOME	DATA INDICATING THAT OUTCOME IS REACHED
Renal tissue perfusion is adequate.	Renal function tests are normal or stable.
Fluid balance is normal.	Urine volume is normal and balances intake; there is no sign of edema.
Nutritional status is normal.	No restrictions are required on food or fluids.

→ › ›

PATIENT OUTCOME	DATA INDICATING THAT OUTCOME IS REACHED
No infection is present.	No signs or symptoms of infection are noted.
There is no alteration in patient's thought processes or response to sensory or perceptual stimuli.	Patient is oriented to time, place, and person.
Patient has resumed self-care.	Patient has no restrictions in activities of daily living (ADL).
Family has adapted to patient's illness and recovery.	The family has dealt with the crisis constructively and can identify sources of help available.
Patient and family are knowledgeable about ARF.	Patient and family can explain ARF, its causes, manifestations, and treatment; the need for medical follow-up; and the potential need for dialysis or transplantation in the future.

PATIENT TEACHING

1. Explain the cause of the episode of acute renal failure.
2. Explain the level of renal function after the acute phase is over.
3. Explain diet and fluid restrictions, which may continue or may be lessened or discontinued.
4. Teach self-observational skills such as measuring temperature, pulse, respirations, blood pressure, intake and output, daily weight, and record keeping.
5. Explain good personal hygiene.
6. Explain how to avoid infections.
7. Explain exercise and rest in the amounts advised.
8. Describe medications, if any, with name, purpose, dosage, time interval, and adverse reactions (by discussion and in writing).
9. Explain the schedule of medical follow-up.
10. Explain renal dialysis and transplantation if they are likely options for the future.

Chronic Renal Failure

Chronic renal failure (CRF) is a slow, insidious, and irreversible impairment of renal function. Uremia usually develops slowly.

Major causes of CRF include polycystic kidney disease, chronic glomerulonephritis, chronic pyelonephritis, chronic urinary obstruction, hypertensive nephropathy, diabetic nephropathy, and gouty nephropathy. These causes can arise as primary renal disease or secondary to other systemic diseases. Primary renal disease includes glomerulonephritis, pyelonephritis, polycystic kidneys, and renal cell carcinoma. Causes that develop secondary to systemic disease include hypertensive nephropathy, diabetic nephropathy, gouty nephropathy, lupus nephritis, renal amyloidosis, myeloma kidney, nephrocalcinosis, and hereditary nephropathy.

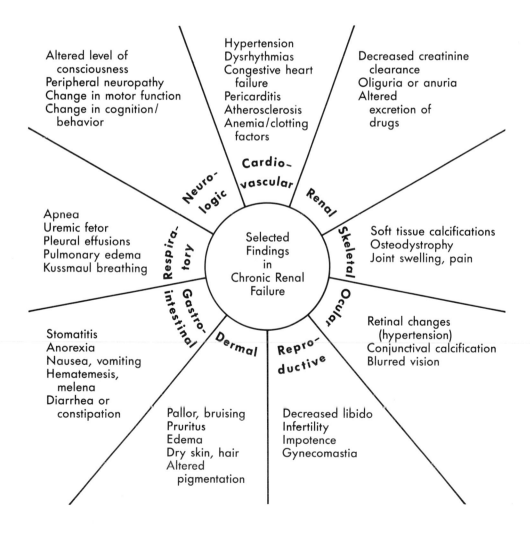

Altered level of
  consciousness
Peripheral neuropathy
Change in motor function
Change in cognition/
  behavior

Hypertension
Dysrhythmias
Congestive heart
  failure
Pericarditis
Atherosclerosis
Anemia/clotting
  factors

Decreased creatinine
  clearance
Oliguria or anuria
Altered
  excretion of
  drugs

Neuro-logic · **Cardio-vascular** · **Renal**

Apnea
Uremic fetor
Pleural effusions
Pulmonary edema
Kussmaul breathing

Respiratory · **Skeletal**

Soft tissue calcifications
Osteodystrophy
Joint swelling, pain

Selected
Findings
in
Chronic Renal
Failure

Gastro-intestinal · **Dermal** · **Reproductive** · **Ocular**

Stomatitis
Anorexia
Nausea, vomiting
Hematemesis,
  melena
Diarrhea or
  constipation

Retinal changes
  (hypertension)
Conjunctival calcification
Blurred vision

Pallor, bruising
Pruritus
Edema
Dry skin, hair
Altered
  pigmentation

Decreased libido
Infertility
Impotence
Gynecomastia

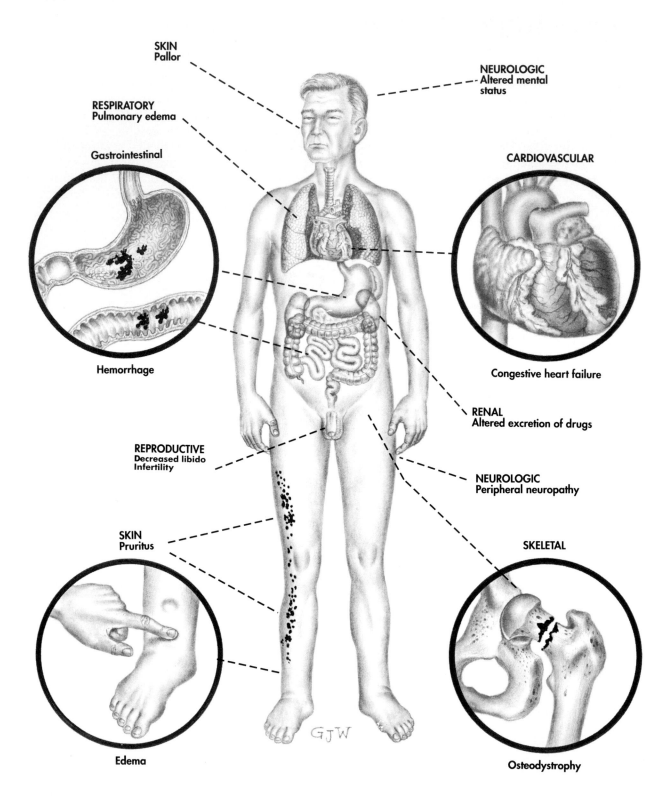

SKIN
Pallor

NEUROLOGIC
Altered mental
status

RESPIRATORY
Pulmonary edema

CARDIOVASCULAR

Gastrointestinal

Hemorrhage

Congestive heart failure

RENAL
Altered excretion of drugs

REPRODUCTIVE
Decreased libido
Infertility

NEUROLOGIC
Peripheral neuropathy

SKIN
Pruritus

SKELETAL

Edema

Osteodystrophy

CHRONIC RENAL FAILURE

The levels of chronic renal failure are identified by changes in the glomerular filtration rate (GFR). In early renal failure, the rate is 30 to 10 ml per minute; in late renal failure, it is 10 to 5 ml per minute; in the terminal stage, it is 5 ml per minute. Symptoms are prominent in later renal failure and life threatening in terminal renal failure or end-stage renal disease (ESRD) (see box). Because patients vary greatly in their clinical picture, renal function, and performance capabilities, the Renal Section of the Council on Circulation of the American Heart Association developed criteria for evaluating the severity of established renal disease.[7] These criteria take into account the severity of the signs and symptoms, the level of impairment of renal function (GFR and serum creatinine), and the performance level (what the patient says she can do).

PATHOPHYSIOLOGY

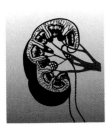

The various causes of failing renal function eventually lead to a final common pathway. Often the specific, initial renal insult cannot be identified.

When the kidneys fail, a variety of substances accumulate that normally are excreted. These substances include nitrogenous wastes, the so-called uremic toxins, and normal substances such as electrolytes that may alter cellular function (i.e., enzyme pathways).

A variety of pathogenic processes can cause chronic renal failure. Infections, for example, may be localized or may accompany systemic disease. Autoimmune disorders may be caused by antigen-antibody complexes and antiglomerular basement membrane antibodies. Metabolic disorders such as renal tubular acidosis and calcium-phosphate abnormalities may cause renal calculi (Table 4-1). Renovascular changes may arise from occlusion, stenosis or thrombosis, diabetes mellitus, or hypertension. Urinary obstruction, renal cancer, and congenital anomalies all may end in chronic renal failure. These topics are discussed in some detail in later chapters.

Nephrons are permanently destroyed by various processes that occur in the course of renal disease, such as ischemia, inflammation, necrosis, fibrosis, sclerosis, and scarring. The normal nephrons remaining may respond with hypertrophy and hyperplasia. Eventually a point is reached when renal deficits become manifest, although as many as 50% of the nephrons may be lost before these deficits are discovered. Such deficits include the inability to respond to excessive salt intake or decreased water or salt intake, decreased synthesis of substances such as erythropoietin by the kidneys, and

> ### SIGNS AND SYMPTOMS OF END-STAGE RENAL DISEASE (UREMIC SYNDROME)
>
> - "Restless legs" and burning sensation of soles of feet
> - Apathy
> - Confusion
> - Stupor
> - Flapping tremor of hands (asterixis)
> - Insomnia
> - Anorexia
> - Nausea and vomiting
> - Uremic fetor (breath odor)
> - Melena
> - Dyspnea
> - Crackles on auscultation of lungs
> - Cardiac dysrhythmias
> - Pericardial rub on auscultation
> - Additional heart sounds (fluid overload)
> - Cardiomegaly
> - Edema (dependent areas)
> - Poor skin turgor (generalized)
> - Pruritis
> - Brittle nails and hair
> - Anemia (normocytic, normochromic)
> - Easy bruising
> - Bleeding (gums, nose, GI tract)
> - Oliguria or anuria
>
> From Thelan.[26]

inability to excrete the end products of metabolism. All the organ systems are eventually affected by renal dysfunction (Table 4-2).

Changes in renal function may be manifested by an increase or decrease in substances usually found in the body (e.g., hemoglobin, blood urea nitrogen, serum creatinine, sodium, calcium, phosphate, and potassium). The body's attempts to accommodate these changes may cause hypertension; pulmonary edema; altered protein, carbohydrate, and fat metabolism; and osteodystrophy. Mental status, peripheral nerve conduction time, and platelet adhesiveness also may be altered.

COMPLICATIONS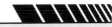

Anemia	Accelerated atherosclerosis
Hypertension	Bleeding diathesis
Hyperkalemia	Peptic ulcer disease
Congestive heart failure	Osteodystrophy
Pulmonary edema	Metabolic encephalopathy
Pericarditis	Peripheral neuropathy

Table 4-1_____

CALCIUM AND PHOSPHATE METABOLISM IN CHRONIC RENAL FAILURE

Kidney	Plasma	Bone
Loss of nephron mass Decreased GFR Decreased phosphate excretion	Elevated phosphate Formation of $CaPO_4$ Decreased ionized calcium	
Increased phosphate excretion (phosphaturia)	Increased PTH secretion (secondary hyperparathyroidism)	Release of calcium and phosphate
Increased calcium reabsorption and increased vitamin D formation (increased intestinal absorption of calcium)	Increased calcium	Osteitis fibrosa, osteomalacia, calcium deposits in soft tissure (occurs when kidney fails to respond to PTH secretion because of loss of renal mass and calcium and phosphate continue to be absorbed from bone)

From McCance.[16]

Table 4-2_____

SYSTEMIC EFFECTS OF UREMIA

System	Manifestations	Mechanisms	Treatment
Skeletal	Osteitis fibrosa (bone inflammation with fibrous degeneration); bone demineralization (principally subperiosteal loss of cortical bone in the fibers, lateral ends of the clavicles, and lamina dura of the teeth); spontaneous fractures, bone pain, osteomalacia (rickets) with end-stage renal failure	Bone resorption associated with hyperparathyroidism, vitamin D deficiency, and demineralization; lowered calcium and raised phosphate levels	Control of hyperphosphatemia to reduced hyperparathyroidism; administration of calcium and aluminum hydroxide antacids, which bind phosphate in the gut, together with a phosphate-restricted diet; vitamin D replacement; avoidance of magnesium antacids because of impaired magnesium excretion
Cardiopulmonary	Hypertension; pericarditis with fever, chest pain, and pericardial friction rub; pulmonary edema; Kussmaul's respirations	Extracellullar volume expansion as cause of hypertension; hypersecretion of renin also associated with hypertension; fluid overload associated with pulmonary edema; and acidosis leading to Kussmaul's respirations	Volume reduction with diuretics that are not potassium sparing (to avoid hyperkalemia); combination of propranolol, hydralazine, and minoxidil for those with high levels of renin; bilateral nephrectomy with dialysis or transplantation
Neurologic	Encephalopathy (fatigue, loss of attention, difficulty problem solving); peripheral neuropathy (pain and burning in the legs and feet, loss of vibration sense and deep tendon reflexes); loss of motor coordination, twitching, fasciculations; stupor and coma with advanced uremia	Uremic toxins associated with end-stage renal disease	Dialysis

DIAGNOSTIC STUDIES AND FINDINGS

Diagnostic test	Findings
Laboratory tests	
Urinalysis	pH: acidic; osmolality: low; specific gravity: fixed; sediment: may contain WBCs, RBCs, and granular, hyaline, broad, and waxy casts; 24-hr volume decreased or nonexistent; proteinuria
Complete blood count	Hgb/Hct lowered; decreased RBC survival time; platelets reduced in number with decreased adhesiveness
Blood chemistry	Decreased serum pH, bicarbonate, and magnesium; increased potassium, sodium, hydrogen, phosphate, and calcium ions; increased serum uric acid, osmolality, BUN; decreased iron and total iron-binding capacity
Creatinine clearance	Decreased
Kidney-ureter-bladder (KUB) x-ray	Small, contracted kidneys
Renal ultrasound	Small, contracted kidneys

Table 4-2

SYSTEMIC EFFECTS OF UREMIA—cont'd

System	Manifestations	Mechanisms	Treatment
Hematologic	Anemia, usually normochromic normocytic, platelet disorders with prolonged bleeding times	Reduced erythropoietin secretion associated with loss of renal mass, leading to reduced red cell production in the bone marrow; uremic toxins associated with shortened red cell survival	Dialysis
Gastrointestinal	Anorexia, nausea, vomiting; mouth ulcers, stomatitis, urinous breath (uremic fetor); hiccups; peptic ulcers; gastrointestinal bleeding; and pancreatitis associated with end-stage renal failure	Retention of metabolic acids and other metabolic waste products	Protein-restricted diet for relief of nausea and vomiting
Integumentary	Abnormal pigmentation and pruritus	Retention of urochromes contributing to sallow, yellow color; high plasma calcium levels associated with pruritus	Dialysis with control of serum calcium levels
Immunologic	Increased risk of infection that can cause death	Suppression of cell-mediated immunity; reduction in number and function of lymphocytes, diminished phagocytosis	Routine dialysis
Reproductive	Sexual dysfunction. menorrhagia, amenorrhea, infertility, and decreased libido in women; decreased testosterone levels, infertility, and decreased libido in men	Probably related to dysfunction of ovaries and testes	No specific treatment

(From McCance.[16])

MEDICAL MANAGEMENT

GENERAL MANAGEMENT

Conservative management of CRF is initiated when marked decreases in renal function are noted and is continued until the need for dialysis or transplantation is determined. The principles guiding management are (1) treat underlying renal disease, (2) prolong the life of the native kidneys, (3) identify and prevent causes of ARF in the presence of CRF, (4) treat the complications of CRF, and (5) relieve the symptoms of uremia.

The goal is to maintain the ideal body weight, which is the weight at which blood pressure is easily controlled without postural hypotension.

Dialysis: peritoneal or hemodialysis (see pages 134 to 152).

Fluid intake should balance output: about 400-600 ml (about the amount of insensible losses) plus an amount equal to 24-hr urine volume; avoid dehydration and volume excess.

Diet modifications focus on providing vitamins and controlling the intake of protein, carbohydrates, fat, sodium, potassium, and phosphate. A high-protein diet increases renal blood flow and GFR and appears to accelerate the natural deterioration of renal function in patients with a variety of kidney lesions. This finding is the basis for using a low-protein diet early in the course of renal disease.

Other nutritional modifications are made to achieve or maintain adequate nutritional status and to reduce the work of the diseased kidneys:

Protein: 0.6 g/kg body weight/day; GFR 20-25 ml/min-90 g/day; GFR 10-15 ml/min-50 g/day; GFR 4-10 ml/min-40 g/day.

Sodium: 1,000-2,000 mg/day; the specific amount depends on weight, blood pressure, serum creatinine, and 24-hr urine sodium excretion.

Potassium: 1,500-2,000 mg/day; no restriction is needed with normal urine output (at least 800 ml/day).

Calories: 35-55 kcal/kg body weight; calories from fat and carbohydrates are used; adequate calories must accompany protein intake to prevent the use of protein for energy and weight loss.

Vitamins: B complex, B_{12} C, folic acid, and D.

DRUG THERAPY

Alkalinizing agents: Sodium bicarbonate, sodium citrate and citric acid (Shohl's Solution).

Potassium-lowering agents: Sodium polystyrene sulfonate (Kayexalate), calcium gluconate, sodium bicarbonate, 50% glucose and regular insulin.

Anticonvulsants: Phenytoin (Dilantin), diazepam (Valium), phenobarbital (Luminal and others).

Antihypertensives: Clonidine (Catapres), diazoxide (Hyperstat IV), hydralazine (Apresoline), methyldopa (Aldomet), prazosin (Minipress), propranolol (Inderal), captopril (Capoten).

Diuretics: Furosemide (Lasix).

Antiinfective agents: Infection is frequently a complication of chronic renal failure; agents specific to the microorganism cultured should be used.

NOTE: Agents whose route of excretion is primarily renal should be omitted or used in smaller doses or at lengthened intervals, depending on the GFR; agents excreted by the liver only require no change; if partial excretion occurs via the kidneys, some adjustment is needed at lower GFRs.

Phosphate-binding agents: Calcium acetate (PhosLo) and aluminum antacids (which also increase gastric pH).

H_2 receptor blockers: Cimetidine (Tagamet), ranitidine (Zantac).

Anabolic agents: Fluoxymesterone (Halotestin), methandrostenolone (Dianabol), nandrolone decanoate (Deca-Durabolin).

Antianemics: Recombinant human erythropoietin (r-hEPO) (Epogen). *Initial dose:* 50-100 U/kg body weight 3 times/wk; IV administration for dialysis patients, IV or subcutaneous administration for nondialysis CRF patients. Maintenance doses are individually titrated.

MEDICAL MANAGEMENT—cont'd

Antiemetics: Prochlorperazine (Compazine), trimethobenzamide (Tigan).

Antipruritics: Cyproheptadine (Periactin), trimeprazine (Temaril).

Laxatives/stool softeners: Methylcellulose (Methulose), docusate sodium (Colace).

Electrolytes/minerals: Calcium carbonate, ferrous sulfate, iron-dextran injection (Imferon).

Vitamins: Thiamine, riboflavin, niacin, pantothenic acid, pyridoxine, vitamin B_{12}, vitamin C, folic acid, vitamin D (calcitriol, dihydrotachysterol).

SURGERY

Renal transplantation (page 157); creation of an internal arteriovenous fistula for hemodialysis or insertion of a Tenckhoff catheter for peritoneal dialysis.

1 ASSESS

ASSESSMENT	OBSERVATIONS
Renal	Oliguria, anuria; infection (WBCs, bacteria); urine sediment may contain RBCs and granular, hyaline, and broad, waxy casts; decreased creatinine clearance
Cardiovascular	Edema; hypertension; anemia (normochromic, normocytic); congestive heart failure; pericarditis; dysrhythmias; cardiomegaly; atherosclerosis
Dermatologic	Pruritus; excoriations; yellow-tan or grayish color; uremic frost; pallor; bruises; fragile, dry skin; thin, brittle nails
Electrolytes	Increased potassium, hydrogen, sodium, phosphate, and magnesium; decreased bicarbonate and calcium
Gastrointestinal	Urinelike odor on breath; metallic taste; stomatitis and gingivitis; loss of sense of smell; anorexia; nausea; vomiting and hematemesis; esophagitis; gastritis; hiccoughs; melena; diarrhea or constipation; thirst
Metabolic	Increased BUN and serum creatinine levels; increased uric acid level; anion gap greater than 9-13 mEq/L; carbohydrate intolerance and altered glucose tolerance curve (delayed rate of decrease); altered insulin degradation (decreased renal extraction); hypertriglyceridemia (impaired removal of triglycerides by lipoprotein lipase activity); acidosis; tetany
Neurologic	Changes in cognitive function and behavior; altered levels of consciousness (drowsiness to coma and convulsions); changes in motor function and proprioception; peripheral neuropathy; nocturnal leg cramping; formication and other paresthesias of lower extremities; apathy, lethargy, and fatigue; headaches; insomnia
Ocular	Retinal changes (hypertension); "red eyes" (calcification of conjunctiva); blurred vision

ASSESSMENT	OBSERVATIONS
Reproductive	Infertility; impotence; amenorrhea; decreased libido; gynecomastia
Respiratory	Pulmonary edema; pneumonia; pleural effusions; hyperventilation; Kussmaul breathing; apnea
Skeletal	Renal osteodystrophy; soft tissue calcification; fractures; bone pain; increased alkaline phosphatase; joint swelling and pain
General	Weight loss

2   DIAGNOSE

NURSING DIAGNOSIS	SUBJECTIVE FINDINGS	OBJECTIVE FINDINGS
Altered renal tissue perfusion related to nephron destruction with inability to excrete metabolic wastes	None	Oliguria, anuria; acidosis with increased serum hydrogen and potassium; decreased bicarbonate, pH; anemia; increased BUN, serum creatinine; decreased calcium and increased phosphate and magnesium
Fluid volume excess related to inability to excrete sodium and water	Describes dyspnea, anxiety, and change in mental status	Hypertension; ascites; presacral and pretibial edema; altered breath sounds (crackles); tachycardia; weight gain; orthopnea; increased central venous pressure and pulmonary artery wedge pressure, jugular venous distention; positive hepatojugular reflex
Altered nutrition: less than body requirements related to restricted dietary intake and gastrointestinal effects of uremia, which result primarily in protein-calorie malnutrition	Complains of anorexia, nausea, and indigestion; dry, sore mouth; metallic taste; thirst; weakness and fatigue	Vomiting, diarrhea, melena, hematemesis, urinelike odor to breath, stomatitis, gingivitis, weight loss
Potential for infection related to suppressed immune responses associated with uremia	None	Signs and symptoms of infection in body secretions, excretions, exudates; fever, chills; increased WBC; positive cultures of urine, blood, and sputum
Potential for impaired skin integrity related to effects of uremia	Complains of pruritus	Petechiae, purpura, dry skin, excoriations

NURSING DIAGNOSIS	SUBJECTIVE FINDINGS	OBJECTIVE FINDINGS
Potential for sensory/perceptual alterations, altered thought processes related to endogenous chemical abnormalities associated with uremia	Reports decreased ability to concentrate, problems with coordination, insomnia, memory loss, emotional lability	Disorientation to time, place, or person; behavior changes, apathy, anger; altered sleep patterns; altered level of consciousness: somnolence, coma; seizures
Potential for bathing/hygiene, toileting self-care deficit related to side effects of uremia	Complains of weakness, fatigue	None
Potential for sexual dysfunction related to effects of uremia	Complains of decreased libido, impotence, erectile difficulties	Menses cease; gynecomastia
Potential for body image disturbance related to permanent alteration of renal function	Expresses disbelief, fear of others' rejection, anxiety, discouragement, resentment, irritability	Denies reality of situation; demonstrates changes in social interaction; aggressive behavior
Potential for altered family processes related to chronic renal failure of family member	Expresses inability to adapt to or deal with family member's illness	Family members may avoid visiting patient or interacting with physician and nurse; may not make use of resources offered, such as chaplain or social worker

3 PLAN

Patient goals

1. The patient will demonstrate a stable level of renal function.
2. The patient will demonstrate a balance between fluid intake and losses.
3. The patient will demonstrate adequate nutritional intake within the restrictions necessary.
4. The patient will be free of infection.
5. The patient will have no impairment of skin integrity.
6. The patient will demonstrate normal responses to sensory and perceptual stimuli and normal thought processes.
7. The patient will resume activities of daily living.
8. The patient will demonstrate acceptance of altered sexuality.
9. The patient will demonstrate adaptation to the change in body image associated with chronic renal failure.
10. The family will demonstrate adaptation to the patient's disorder.
11. The patient will demonstrate increased knowledge of chronic renal failure, its cause, manifestations, and treatment; the need for medical follow-up; and the potential need for dialysis or transplantation.

4 IMPLEMENT

NURSING DIAGNOSIS	NURSING INTERVENTIONS	RATIONALE
Altered renal tissue perfusion related to nephron destruction with inability to excrete metabolic wastes	Assess ECG for changes, respirations (rate and depth), Chvostek's and Trousseau's signs.	Peaked T wave, prolonged PR interval and widened QRS complex are associated with increased serum potassium; Kussmaul respirations are associated with acidosis; tetany may occur with low calcium level.
	Monitor laboratory data: serum pH, hydrogen, potassium, bicarbonate; calcium, magnesium, phosphate; hemoglobin, hematocrit; blood urea nitrogen, serum creatinine.	Levels reflect kidneys' ability to excrete nitrogenous wastes, excess fluids, and electrolytes; values also indicate kidney's nonexcretory functions (e.g., erythropoietin production).
	Avoid nephrotoxic drugs.	Ability to excrete drugs normally removed by the kidneys is reduced.
	Administer medications as ordered with care; monitor response to drugs.	Doses of medications may be less than usual, and intervals between doses may be lengthened; monitoring determines the effectiveness of drug, dosage, and timing and aids in identifying adverse side effects.
Fluid volume excess related to inability to excrete sodium and water	Assess weight daily, also 24-h intake and output; assess blood pressure (standing and sitting), pulse and respirations (including breath sounds) q 6-8 h; assess mental status; monitor edema, jugular venous distention, hepatojugular reflex and, if necessary, central venous pressure and pulmonary artery wedge pressure.	To identify altered fluid status.
	Monitor laboratory data: serum sodium, potassium, chloride, bicarbonate.	To identify electrolyte accumulations.
	Monitor ECG.	Increase or decrease in potassium may be associated with dysrhythmias; potassium may be lowered by vigorous diuretic therapy.
	Offer limited fluid intake over 24 hr; cool liquids may help quench thirst. Provide mouth care.	To avoid nocturnal dehydration, since the kidneys' normal diurnal variation in urine output is lost.
	Administer diuretics as ordered; monitor response.	To determine the effect of drugs and observe for side effects such as hypokalemia and ototoxicity.

NURSING DIAGNOSIS	NURSING INTERVENTIONS	RATIONALE
Altered nutrition: less than body requirements related to restricted dietary intake and gastrointestinal effects of uremia, which cause primarily protein-calorie malnutrition	Assess for nausea, vomiting, and anorexia.	These conditions increase losses of needed nutrients.
	Monitor food intake and dry weight; monitor laboratory data: serum protein, lipids, potassium, and sodium.	To determine how well the diet is being followed.
	Encourage food intake as prescribed; postpone meals, if necessary; serve food the patient likes, and present it attractively.	To ensure adequate intake within limits prescribed.
	Provide oral hygiene before meals; offer sour candy and gum.	To help remove bad taste in mouth.
	Administer antiemetics, and monitor response.	To determine the effect of dose and timing and to observe for adverse side effects.
	Refer complex or problem situations to dietitian.	A team approach to managing the complex renal diet is helpful to all concerned.
Potential for infection related to suppressed immune responses associated with uremia	Assess for signs and symptoms of infection in secretions, excretions, exudates; assess for fever and chills.	To detect any infection early.
	Monitor temperature q 4-6 hr; monitor laboratory data: WBC; blood, urine, and sputum cultures; serum potassium.	Uremia may mask the usual increase in temperature found with infection; a hypermetabolic state such as infection can cause a marked rise in serum potassium.
	Wash hands thoroughly and consistently; avoid exposing patient to people with infection; ensure aseptic technique for any invasive procedure or wound care.	To decrease chances of infection.
	Encourage regular oral hygiene, hand washing, bathing, adequate nutrition, and rest.	Good health habits help prevent infection.
Potential for impaired skin integrity related to effects of uremia	Assess for dry skin, pruritus, excoriations, and infection.	Changes may be related to decreased activity of sweat glands or deposits of calcium or phosphate crystals in cutaneous layers.
	Assess for petechiae and purpura.	Bleeding abnormalities are related to decreased number and altered function of platelets in uremia.
	Monitor skin folds and edematous areas.	These areas are easily injured.
	Provide meticulous care to normal and injured areas of skin.	To prevent injury and infection and to help healing.

NURSING DIAGNOSIS	NURSING INTERVENTIONS	RATIONALE
	Administer antipruritic drugs; vinegar or starch baths; use bland soap sparingly.	To relieve pruritus.
	Keep fingernails trimmed.	To decrease injury during scratching.
Potential for sensory/perceptual alterations; altered thought processes related to endogenous chemical abnormalities associated with uremia	Assess neurologic status; orientation to person, place, and time; sleep pattern; level of consciousness; and seizure activity.	Changes reflect alterations in central and autonomic nervous system function.
	Assess premorbid personality.	To identify changes associated with uremia.
	Observe for changes in behavior and presence of peripheral neuropathy: restless legs, burning feet, muscle cramps, other paresthesias, dysesthesias.	Metabolic changes may cause cerebral dysfunction; demyelination of large nerve fibers and axonal degeneration may occur.
	Orient patient to reality.	To decrease possibility that disorientation is due to isolation and lack of information.
	Maintain safety precautions: bed rails up, bed in low position, sharp objects out of reach, call bell in reach; institute seizure precautions if needed.	To provide safe environment and prevent injury.
	Allow extra time for patient to respond to questions and to process new information. Use a consistent, calm, nonargumentative approach.	Short-term memory loss may occur.
	Encourage normal daytime activities and presleep relaxation training; provide periods of rest.	To maintain or encourage normal sleep-rest patterns; uremia can reverse sleep-wake patterns.
Potential for bathing/hygiene, toileting self-care deficit related to uremia	Assess fatigue and weakness, and assist with care as needed.	To determine assistance needed.
	Implement measures such as deep breathing, coughing, and turning regularly.	To prevent adverse effects of bed rest, such as pneumonia.
	Increase activity as tolerated.	To help patient return to self-care as appropriate.
Potential for sexual dysfunction related to effects of uremia	Assess patient-spouse response to alterations.	To determine presence of problems.
	Allow patient and spouse to talk about their feelings; suggest positive aspects of closeness and touching without intercourse.	To help patient and spouse adjust to changes.
	Refer patient and spouse for counseling when needed.	To help resolve problems requiring time and skills beyond the nurse's capability.

NURSING DIAGNOSIS	NURSING INTERVENTIONS	RATIONALE
Potential for body image disturbance related to altered renal function	Assess for evidence that change in renal function or in appearance or the possibility of dialysis or transplantation is a problem; allow patient to talk about his feelings; recognize defense mechanisms such as denial, guilt, aggression, fear, displacement, regression, resentment, disbelief, and anxiety; recognize losses in psychosocial aspects of patient's life; isolation, job loss, financial instability, dependency, and altered hopes for the future may be problems.	Early intervention may prevent patient distress.
	Explain skin changes to patient (in color, easy bruising).	Pallor may be due to anemia, yellowish cast to urochrome pigment deposits in skin; blacks become more deeply pigmented, and Hispanics and Asians show pallor.
	Offer emotional support; refer to other professional services if needed.	To increase patient's acceptance of condition.
Potential for altered family processes related to CRF of family member	Assess family structure and role relationships.	To identify family strengths.
	Monitor family's response to illness, treatment, and prognosis.	To identify potential problems.
	Encourage patient and family members to discuss their needs and concerns; discuss impact of situation on roles and adaptation required.	To help in adjustments indicated.
	Assist with problem solving, and support family decisions.	Crisis intervention may be needed.
	Refer to other services as appropriate.	To help resolve problems requiring time and skills beyond the nurse's capability.
Knowledge deficit	See Patient Teaching.	

5 EVALUATE

PATIENT OUTCOME	DATA INDICATING THAT OUTCOME IS REACHED
Renal tissue perfusion is adequate.	Renal function tests are normal or stable.
Fluid balance is normal.	Urine output balances intake; there are no or minimum signs of edema.

→ > >

PATIENT OUTCOME	DATA INDICATING THAT OUTCOME IS REACHED
Patient's nutritional status has improved and is maintained.	Food and fluid intakes are within the limits imposed by CRF; dry weight is maintained or increased if necessary.
No infection is present.	No signs or symptoms of infection are noted.
Skin is intact.	Patient has no areas of excoriation.
Thought processes and responses to sensory and perceptual stimuli are normal or stable.	Patient is oriented to time, place, and person; alterations in sensation are not progressing; sleep pattern is normal.
Patient has resumed self-care.	Patient has no or few restrictions in ADL.
Patient has accepted alterations in sexuality.	Patient has acceptable sexual relationships within the limits imposed by CRF.
Patient has adapted to changes in body image associated with CRF.	Patient demonstrates adjustment to altered renal function and any change in appearance.
Patient and family have adapted to patient's disorder.	Patient and family have dealt constructively with diagnosis and treatment regimen and can identify available sources of help.
Patient and family are knowledgeable about CRF.	Patient and family can explain CRF, its causes and manifestations; the need for medical follow-up; and the potential need for dialysis or transplantation in the future.

PATIENT TEACHING

1. Explain the nature of chronic renal failure.
2. Explain the medical regimen and its rationale, including diet (restricted protein, sodium, and potassium intake), restricted fluid intake, and medications (purpose, dosage, interval, and adverse reactions).
3. Teach the patient self-observational skills (temperature, pulse, respirations, blood pressure, intake and output, and weight) and record keeping.
4. Explain avoidance of infection.
5. Explain personal hygiene, rest, and exercise.
6. Explain when to call the physician.
7. Explain the plan for medical follow-up.
8. Explain renal dialysis and transplantation.

CHAPTER 5

Infectious Diseases

Pyelonephritis

Pyelonephritis (PLN) is an infection of the kidney and renal pelvis. It is a major problem of the renal system.

Pyelonephritis is one of a group of conditions generally called **urinary tract infections** (the others are asymptomatic **bacteriuria** and **cystitis**). Urinary tract infections occur more frequently in women than in men, and the incidence of such infections increases with age, instrumentation of the urinary tract, and urologic abnormalities, including vesicoureteral reflux or urinary tract obstruction (Table 5-1).

Although urinary tract infections, including PLN, cause considerable morbidity, they do not progress to end-stage renal disease unless there is an underlying urinary tract problem such as obstruction. During pregnancy women should be screened for bacteriuria and treated to prevent the development of PLN. Personal health habits should include adequate fluid intake (2,500-3,000 ml/day) and prompt emptying of the bladder.

PATHOPHYSIOLOGY

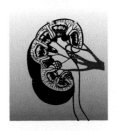

The infection in PLN is caused by bacteria that spread by hematogenous or lymphatic routes or most commonly by ascending from the lower urinary tract. The organisms most frequently involved are gram-negative bacilli and enterococci, bacteria that colonize the bowel.

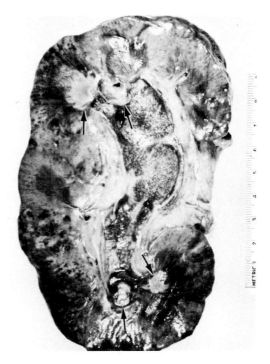

FIGURE 5-1
Papillary necrosis resulting from acute pyelonephritis and obstruction. Note necrotic papillae *(arrows)*, mottled patchy cortical infiltrate of acute pyelonephritis, and congested, dilated renal pelvis. (From Kissane.[13])

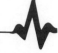

Table 5-1

COMMON CAUSES OF PYELONEPHRITIS

Predisposing	Pathologic mechanisms
Kidney stones	Obstruction and stasis of urine contributing to bacteriuria and hydronephrosis; irritation of epithelial lining with entrapment of bacteria
Vesicoureteral reflux	Chronic reflux of urine up the ureter and into kidney during micturition contributing to bacterial infection
Pregnancy	Dilation and relaxation of ureter with hydroureter and hydronephrosis; partly caused by obstruction from enlarged uterus and partly from ureteral relaxation caused by higher progesterone levels
Neurogenic bladder	Neurologic impairment interfering with normal bladder contraction with residual urine and ascending infection
Instrumentation	Introduction of organisms into urethra and bladder by catheters and endoscopes introduced into the urinary tract for diagnostic purposes
Female sexual trauma	Movement of organisms from the urethra into the bladder with infection and retrograde spread to kidney

(From McCance.[16])

They can proliferate in the urine and ascend to the kidneys. *Escherichia coli, Klebsiella pneumoniae, Proteus mirabilis* or *Proteus vulgaris, Pseudomonas aeruginosa,* and *Streptococcus faecalis* all can cause urinary tract infection and progress to PLN.

Obstructive uropathy, glomerulonephritis, polycystic kidney disease, diabetes mellitus, renal calculi, and analgesic abuse appear to lower the kidneys' resistance to infection. Without treatment, a significant number of pregnant women with asymptomatic bacteriuria will develop PLN.

The kidneys are damaged by the inflammation, fibrosis, and scarring caused by the infection. Chronic PLN causes tissue destruction and results in contracted, small kidneys. The medulla is susceptible to the ascending spread of bacteria because of its hypertonic environment and slow blood flow. Infection spreads through the collecting ducts to the interstitium. Papillary necrosis may develop as a complication of PLN, and detached pieces of tissue may block the ureters. Infection spreads to the cortex and eventually involves the nephron and blood vessels. Renal abscesses also may develop (see page 68).

Most infections are acute, although a long-term, smoldering, chronic infection occasionally may occur. One or more of the factors previously mentioned contribute most often to a chronic kidney infection.

COMPLICATIONS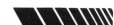

Papillary necrosis (Figure 5-1)
Septicemia

MEDICAL MANAGEMENT

GENERAL MANAGEMENT

The goals of treatment are to eradicate the infection and relieve the symptoms.
High-normal fluid intake (3,500-4,000 ml/day) is prescribed to dilute the urine, decrease burning on urination, flush out the urinary tract, and prevent dehydration (with normal renal function).
Bed rest is common during the acute phase.

DRUG THERAPY

Antiinfective agents: Drugs should be taken for a full 7-10 days; repeat microscopic study of urine and cultures as needed.
(See Table 5-2 for commonly used antimicrobial agents.)

DIAGNOSTIC STUDIES AND FINDINGS

Diagnostic test	Findings
Laboratory tests	
Urinalysis	Antibody-coated bacteria (more often associated with PLN than with cystitis); bacteriuria; WBC casts; pyuria
Complete blood count	Increased WBC
Intravenous urogram	Small kidneys with an irregular outline and focal clubbing of the calyceal system

Table 5-2

ANTIMICROBIAL DRUGS FREQUENTLY USED FOR PYELONEPHRITIS

Parenteral agents	Oral agents
Penicillins	
Penicillin G (Pfizerpen)	Penicillin G (Pentids)
Procaine penicillin G (Wycillin)	
Methicillin (Staphcillin)	Nafcillin (Unipen)
Carbenicillin (Geopen)	Carbenicillin (Geocillin)
Piperacillin (Pipracil)	
Ampicillin (Omnipen)	Ampicillin (Polycillin)
Cephalosporins	
Cefazolin (Ancef, Kefzol)	Cephalexin (Keflex)
Cefoxitin (Mefoxin)	Cefaclor (Ceclor)
Ceftazidime (Fortaz)	Ceftizoxime (Ceftizox)
Aminoglycosides	
Gentamicin (Garamycin)	
Tobramycin (Tobrex)	
Amikacin (Amikin)	
Others	
Co-trimoxazole IV (Septra IV)	Co-trimoxazole (Septra)
	Sulfamethizole (Proklar)
	Sulfisoxazole (Gantrisin)
	Trimethoprim (Proloprim)
	Nalidixic acid (NegGram)
	Norfloxacin (Noroxin)
	Nitrofurantoin (Furadantin)
	Methenamine (Hexamine)

1 ASSESS

ASSESSMENT	OBSERVATIONS
General complaints	Sudden onset of fever, chills
Renal	Hematuria; bacteriuria; pyuria; urine culture: significant growth; dysuria; nocturia; frequency

2 DIAGNOSE

NURSING DIAGNOSIS	SUBJECTIVE FINDINGS	OBJECTIVE FINDINGS
Altered body temperature related to effects of infection	Complains of feeling warm	Fever; chills
Pain (flank) related to distention of renal capsule by infectious process	Reports dull, constant pain in flank	Guarded movements

3 PLAN

Patient goals

1. The patient will have no signs or symptoms of pyelonephritis.

2. The patient will be knowledgeable about the cause of pyelonephritis, its signs and symptoms, treatment, and follow-up medical care.

4 IMPLEMENT

NURSING DIAGNOSIS	NURSING INTERVENTIONS	RATIONALE
Altered body temperature related to effects of infection	Assess for dehydration and diaphoresis. Assess temperature q 4-8 h.	Perspiration is part of the body's attempt to lower temperature; water loss via the skin increases with fever.
	Administer antiinfective agents as ordered, and monitor response; monitor laboratory data: urinalysis and WBC.	To determine effects of drugs and to watch for adverse side effects.
	Encourage bed rest during acute phase of illness.	To increase patient's comfort.
	Encourage high-normal fluid intake unless contraindicated.	To flush kidneys (but avoid lowering drug concentration to ineffective levels).

NURSING DIAGNOSIS	NURSING INTERVENTIONS	RATIONALE
Pain (flank) related to distention of renal capsule by infectious process	Assess need for analgesia; administer analgesics as needed.	As swelling in the kidney decreases, pain lessens; analgesics promote comfort.
	Apply heat externally to painful area.	To help relieve pain.
Knowledge deficit	See Patient Teaching.	

5 EVALUATE

PATIENT OUTCOME	DATA INDICATING THAT OUTCOME IS REACHED
Signs and symptoms of PLN have cleared.	Patient's temperature is normal; pain is gone; urine is clear of bacteria or pus cells; problems in urination are gone.
Evaluation of the urinary tract has been completed.	Intravenous urogram has determined whether there is any structural defect.
Patient is knowledgeable about PLN.	Patient can describe the signs and symptoms of PLN and any further treatment needed.

PATIENT TEACHING

1. Explain pyelonephritis, its causes, signs, and symptoms and the need to have an intravenous urogram to rule out any structural defect.
2. Explain antimicrobial therapy: drugs, dosage, interval, side effects, and the need to complete the course of treatment.
3. Explain the possibility of relapse or reinfection.
4. Explain measures to prevent urinary tract infection: adequate fluid intake (2,000-2,500 ml/day for adults) to avoid dehydration, regular emptying of bladder to avoid overdistention, and good perineal hygiene for women to prevent microorganisms from entering the urinary tract (see page 180.)

Renal and Perinephric Abscesses

A **renal abscess** is a localized infection found within the cortex of the kidney; a **perinephric abscess** is a renal abscess that extends into the tissues around the kidney.

Spread of infection

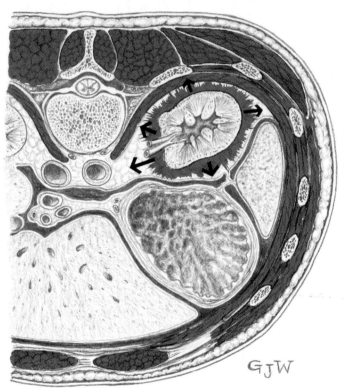

GJW

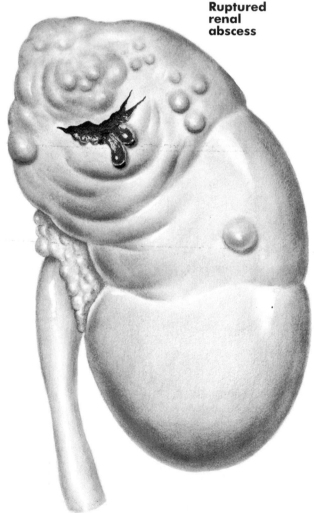

Ruptured renal abscess

Renal abscesses can arise in a normal or diseased kidney; they also can develop as a complication of subacute bacterial endocarditis and systemic infections. With perinephric abscesses, delay in treatment results in a high mortality.

PATHOPHYSIOLOGY

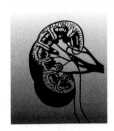

Renal abscesses may be caused by diffuse pyelonephritis or hematogenous transport of bacteria in a systemic infection. Staphylococcal bacteremia, for example, may cause several cortical abscesses. Frequently abscesses are caused by

PREDISPOSING FACTORS FOR RENAL AND PERINEPHRIC ABSCESSES

Ureteral obstruction
Infected renal stones
Diabetes mellitus

For a picture of renal abscess, see Color Plate 2 on page x.

gram-negative organisms such as *Proteus* species and *Escherichia coli*. When infection from the kidney spreads to the fatty and fascial tissues surrounding the kidney, the abscess is known as a perinephric abscess. Drainage collects at the lower pole of the kidney because of the effects of gravity. Such abscesses are frequently associated with renal calculi or urinary tract obstructions. The infection may extend through the fascia to nearby organs such as the pancreas, duodenum, and colon.

COMPLICATIONS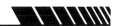

Septicemia

DIAGNOSTIC STUDIES AND FINDINGS

Diagnostic test	Findings
Laboratory test	
White blood cell count	Elevated
Intravenous urogram	Renal mass, calyceal distortion, or renal displacement
Renal computed tomography (CT) scan	Differentiates between an abscess and a cyst

MEDICAL MANAGEMENT

GENERAL MANAGEMENT

Bed rest, adequate fluids (2,500-3,000 ml/day), and normal nutrition are important; a normal diet ensures protein, calories, and other nutrients sufficient to meet the needs of the individual's current stage of the life cycle; sterile dressing changes are needed after incision and drainage of abscesses.

DRUG THERAPY

Antiinfective agents: Sulfisoxazole (Gantrisin), ampicillin (Omnipen), carbenicillin (Geopen), gentamicin (Garamycin).

Antipyretics: For fever, acetaminophen (Tylenol).

SURGERY

Incision and drainage may be required if the renal abscess is localized; incision and drainage are usually required for perinephric abscesses.

Intrarenal: Percutaneous aspiration and instillation of antibiotics; this procedure is less expensive and causes less discomfort than open drainage.

Perinephric: Percutaneous drainage, if possible, although open surgical drainage is more likely; the specimen is sent for culture and sensitivity determinations.

1 ASSESS

ASSESSMENT	OBSERVATIONS
Signs of infection	Renal abscess: None with solitary abscess; otherwise chills; fever; flank tenderness; nausea; vomiting; anorexia; and malaise Perinephric abscess: Chills and fever; increased WBC; dull ache in flank; costovertebral angle tenderness on palpation; mass in flank; abdominal pain with guarding

2 DIAGNOSE

NURSING DIAGNOSIS	SUBJECTIVE FINDINGS	OBJECTIVE FINDINGS
Impaired skin integrity related to percutaneous or open surgical drainage	None	Flank incision
Pain related to drainage of abscess	Describes flank pain	Guarding behavior

3 PLAN

Patient goals

1. The patient's incision will heal.
2. The patient's pain will be alleviated.

3. The patient will be knowledgeable about renal or perinephric abscess, its cause, and treatment.

4 IMPLEMENT

NURSING DIAGNOSIS	NURSING INTERVENTIONS	RATIONALE
Impaired skin integrity related to percutaneous or open surgical drainage	Assess condition of incision and nature and amount of drainage.	To determine extent of healing.
	Monitor temperature q 6-8 h.	Body temperature rises with infection.
	Administer antimicrobial agents as ordered.	Interruption in dosage can permit drug resistance to develop.
	Encourage oral fluids, up to 3 L/day if not contraindicated.	To flush bacteria from urinary tract.
	Change wound dressing using aseptic technique.	To prevent introduction of additional organisms.
	Monitor laboratory data: WBC.	To follow body's response to infection.
Pain related to drainage of abscess	Assess need for pain relief; administer analgesic drug as ordered; monitor response to analgesic.	Incisional pain is not unusual in first 24 hr; analgesic promotes patient's comfort and monitoring determines effectiveness of drug, dosage, and timing.
Knowledge deficit	See Patient Teaching.	

5 EVALUATE

PATIENT OUTCOME	DATA INDICATING THAT OUTCOME IS REACHED
Infection has cleared.	Temperature is in normal range; patient is pain free; WBC is normal.
Incision has healed.	No sign of infection is noted; wound is closed.
Patient is knowledgeable about renal or perinephric abscess.	Patient can describe the cause and treatment of a renal or perinephric abscess.

PATIENT TEACHING

1. Explain the side effects and possible adverse reactions to the pharmacologic agents used.
2. Explain care of the incision, and teach the patient how to change his dressing if necessary.
3. Explain the relationship between perinephric abscesses and pyelonephritis, renal calculi, and urinary tract obstruction.

Genitourinary Tuberculosis

Genitourinary tuberculosis is an infection caused by *Mycobacterium tuberculosis* and can occur in the kidneys and spread to the rest of the genitourinary tract.

Genitourinary tuberculosis is much less common today than in the past; however, 4,350 new cases of extrapulmonary tuberculosis were reported in the United States in 1989. Of these cases, 383 (8.8%) were in the genitourinary system.[4] Prevention is important; about 4% to 9% of people with active pulmonary tuberculosis develop genitourinary involvement.[7] Contact with people with active pulmonary tuberculosis should be avoided, and early diagnosis is important.

Genitourinary tuberculosis often occurs in older people and in immigrants from places with high prevalence rates. Prophylactic care with isoniazid is important for susceptible individuals (e.g., household members of patients with tuberculosis and persons with positive reactions to the tuberculin skin test).

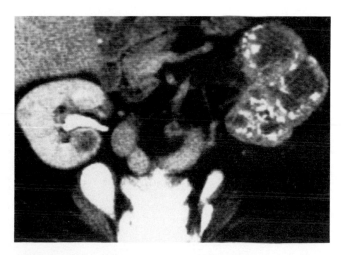

FIGURE 5-2
CT scan of genitourinary tuberculosis. Note mass in posterior portion of right kidney, enlarged left kidney with diffuse calcifications (white areas).

PATHOPHYSIOLOGY

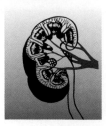

The tuberculosis organism is carried by the bloodstream from the lungs or gastrointestinal tract. Genitourinary tuberculosis is associated with primary pulmonary infection or occurs during reactivation many years later from infection previously seeded in the kidneys. The renal lesion, initially in the glomeruli, causes inflammation, caseation, and rupture, thus spreading the infection to the rest of the nephron and resulting in progressive destruction of the renal parenchyma (Figure 5-2).

Tuberculosis occurs more frequently in men; the bladder, prostate, epididymis, and testicles also may be involved. An abscess in the cortex may erode into a calyx, spreading infection to the pelvis and downward to the bladder. Early treatment of pulmonary tuberculosis may be reducing the number of patients who develop renal lesions.

The tuberculosis organism causes a low-grade inflammation and granuloma formation; healing causes fibrosis, calcification, and scarring, and thus destruction of renal tissue. Damage may obstruct the drainage system and impair the blood supply, causing hypertension.

COMPLICATIONS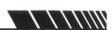

Ureteral strictures
Hydronephrosis
Contracted, noncompliant bladder

DIAGNOSTIC STUDIES AND FINDINGS

Diagnostic test	Findings
Laboratory tests	
Routine urinalysis	Sterile pyuria; hematuria
Early morning urine specimen 3 days in a row	Acid-fast bacillus
Urine culture	*M. tuberculosis* grown
Skin test (intradermal Mantoux)	Positive tuberculin reaction
Intravenous urogram	Cavity formation shown by irregular outline of kidney and calcification; impaired excretion of dye because of parenchymal destruction (tissue may appear "moth eaten"); ureteral stricture; decreased bladder capacity
Kidney-ureter-bladder (KUB) x-ray	Kidney enlarged because of granulomas or hydronephrosis, or shrunken because of fibrosis and atrophy

MEDICAL MANAGEMENT

GENERAL MANAGEMENT

Bed rest may be prescribed at first; ensure adequate nutrition; observe isolation precautions if sputum or urine is positive for tuberculosis bacilli; proper disposal of urine (flushed down toilet, not bedpan flusher) and other infected material (double-bagged and incinerated) is part of the plan of care.

DRUG THERAPY

Antiinfective agents: Rifampin (Rifadin), streptomycin, ethambutol (Etibi), isoniazid (INH).

Vitamin replacement: Pyridoxine for isoniazid-induced deficiency.

SURGERY

May be necessary to remove a nonfunctioning kidney, a continuing source of organisms or uncontrollable hypertension, or other expendable diseased tissues; repair of sequelae, such as ureteral strictures, may be necessary.

1 ASSESS

ASSESSMENT	OBSERVATIONS
General complaints	Fever; weight loss
Urinary tract	Urgency; frequency; flank pain Note: Far-advanced disease may manifest renal failure or urinary tract obstruction; most cases show few or no symptoms

2 DIAGNOSE

NURSING DIAGNOSIS	SUBJECTIVE FINDINGS	OBJECTIVE FINDINGS
Altered renal tissue perfusion related to effects of infection	Reports flank pain	Fever; diaphoresis; weight loss
Altered pattern of urinary elimination related to urinary tract stricture, inflammation	Reports urgency	Frequency
Potential for bathing/hygiene and toileting self-care deficit related to bed rest	Reports lethargy, malaise	Bed rest may be ordered

3 PLAN

Patient goals

1. The patient will demonstrate a normal pattern of renal function.
2. The patient will demonstrate improvement in infection-related symptoms.
3. The patient will resume self-care.
4. The patient will be knowledgeable about genitourinary tuberculosis, its cause, spread, and treatment.

4 IMPLEMENT

NURSING DIAGNOSIS	NURSING INTERVENTIONS	RATIONALE
Altered renal tissue perfusion related to effects of infection	Assess body temperature q 4-8 h.	Body temperature increases during active infection.
	Assess hydration status by examining skin turgor and mucous membrane; provide fluids.	Water loss increases with fever; fluids help maintain normal balance and replace insensible losses.

NURSING DIAGNOSIS	NURSING INTERVENTIONS	RATIONALE
	Administer antimicrobial drugs as ordered.	Interruption in dosage can permit drug resistance to develop.
	Monitor laboratory data: urinalysis, liver function tests.	Acid-fast bacilli should disappear from urine within 2-4 wk of effective therapy; if not, check for drug resistance and compliance; drugs given may alter liver function.
Altered pattern of urinary elimination related to urinary tract stricture, inflammation	Assess frequency and urgency.	Decreased bladder capacity and inflammation of the urinary tract lining cause these symptoms.
	Provide urinal or bedpan.	Patient may not be able to reach toilet in time.
Potential for bathing/hygiene and toileting self-care deficit related to bed rest	Assess patient's compliance; assist with personal hygiene as needed.	Bed rest may be ordered during acute phase of illness.
	Remind patient to turn, cough, breathe deeply, and exercise legs several times a day.	To prevent adverse effects of bed rest such as pneumonia and deep vein thrombosis.
Knowledge deficit	See Patient Teaching.	

5 EVALUATE

PATIENT OUTCOME	DATA INDICATING THAT OUTCOME IS REACHED
Infection has resolved.	Urine culture is negative in 2 mo; temperature is within normal range; follow-up x-ray reveals healing and no strictures.
Pattern of urinary elimination has improved.	Patient experiences no urgency or frequency.
Patient has returned to independent physical activities and self-care.	Patient has no limitations on ADL.
Patient is knowledgeable about genitourinary tuberculosis.	Patient can describe measures to prevent spread of tuberculosis, the rationale for drug treatment, and the side effects of the drugs.

PATIENT TEACHING ■■■■■■■■■■■■■■■■■■■■■■■■■■■■■■■■■■

1. Explain the nature of tuberculosis, its cause, spread, and treatment.

Autoimmune Disorders

Acute Poststreptococcal Glomerulonephritis

Acute poststreptococcal glomerulonephritis (APSGN) is an inflammation of the glomeruli that occurs after a streptococcal infection elsewhere in the body.

Glomerulonephritis can follow a respiratory or skin infection. Several strains of group A beta-hemolytic streptococci that cause GN have been isolated. In temperate zones the most common nephritogenic strain causing pharyngitis is M-type 12. Only about 5% of such infections are followed by APSGN. Children and young adults are affected most frequently. The incidence of APSGN decreases with age, because many children (especially in urban areas) develop immunities to type 12 beta-hemolytic streptococci before reaching adulthood. Renal problems occur abruptly 1 to 3 weeks after the infection. Most patients (95%) recover normal renal function within 2 months. The others have irreversible damage that causes long-term problems. It is not clear whether prompt treatment of streptococcal infections prevents renal complications of APSGN.

PATHOPHYSIOLOGY

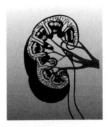

In acute poststreptococcal glomerulonephritis, antibodies of the host react with circulating antigens that appear to arise from the toxic products of the infecting organism; the two form immune complexes that become lodged in the glomeruli (Table 6-1). Both kidneys are affected by an acute, diffuse, nonsuppurative inflammation that damages the glomerular basement membrane (GBM). The kidneys respond through GBM thickening, endocapillary proliferation, scarring, necrosis, and extracapillary proliferation (Figure 6-1). The damage causes an acute interference with renal function. Glomerulonephritis is a very frequent cause of renal failure among patients on dialysis.

COMPLICATIONS

Hypervolemia
Hypertension
Convulsions

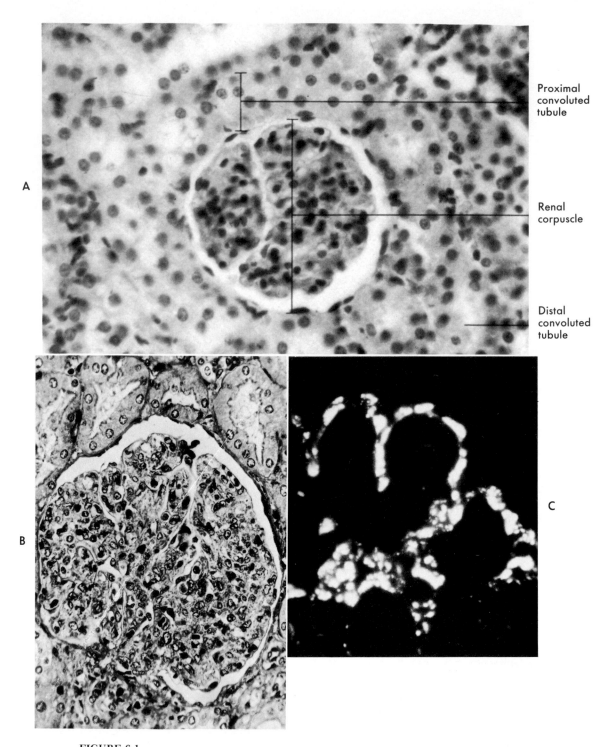

FIGURE 6-1

A, Photomicrograph of kidney showing normal glomerulus surrounded by profiles of sectioned renal tubules (×140). **B,** Acute poststreptococcal glomerulonephritis. Swollen, hypercellular glomerular lobules with few open capillaries. (×250). **C,** Acute poststreptococcal glomerulonephritis. "Humps" of immune complex stained with fluorescent antihuman complement (C3). (×1000). (Courtesy Dr. Caude Cornwall, Syracuse, NY.) (**A** from Thibodeau[26a]; **B** and **C** from Kissane.[13])

Table 6-1

IMMUNOLOGIC PATHOGENESIS OF GLOMERULONEPHRITIS

Glomerular injury	Mechanism
Soluble immune-complex glomerulonephritis (90%)	Formation of antibodies stimulated by the presence of endogenous or exogenous antigens results in circulating soluble antigen-antibody complexes, which are deposited in glomerular capillaries. Glomerular injury occurring with complement activation and release of immunologic substances that lyse cells and increase membrane permeability. Immune deposits with a microscopic appearance that fluoresce in a *granular pattern* when stained with fluorescein and viewed under ultraviolet light. Severity of glomerular injury related to the number of complexes formed.
Antiglomerular basement membrane glomerulonephritis (5%)	Antibodies are formed and act directly against the glomerular basement membrane; immune response that causes crescent formation and a *linear pattern* of immunofluorescence; generally associated with rapidly progressive renal failure such as Goodpasture's syndrome.
Alternative complement pathway	A relatively obscure mechanism associated with low levels of complement and membranoproliferative glomerulonephritis.
Cell-mediated immunity	A delayed hypersensitivity response that damages the glomerulus. Actual cellular mechanism not clearly understood.

(From McCance[16].)

GLOMERULONEPHRITIS

Glomerulonephritis (GN) may be a primary disease of the kidneys or may develop secondary to a systemic disease, such as systemic lupus erythematosus. Glomerulonephritis is a disease primarily of the glomeruli caused by immunologically mediated damage (immune complex or autoantibody). The immune complexes (antibody-antigen) arise from antigens such as those from microorganisms, drugs, and autologous tissues. The major antibody involved is that against the glomerular basement membrane (GBM).

The clinical syndrome may include asymptomatic proteinuria or nephrotic syndrome, microscopic or macroscopic hematuria, or nephritic syndrome. Nephritic syndrome is characterized by moderate proteinuria, normal or slightly decreased serum albumin, minimally decreased plasma lipids, marked hematuria, moderate edema, decreased urine volume and glomerular filtration rate, and hypertension.

Discussion of glomerulonephritis can be difficult because of the confusion between older definitions, used before renal biopsy was introduced, and newer terms used since. One classification of GN uses clinical course (acute, rapidly progressive, and chronic), histopathology (e.g., membranoproliferative), and pathogenetic mechanisms (immune complexes and antibodies against kidney antigens).

The kinds of glomerulonephritis include acute poststreptococcal GN (APSGN) (immune complexes); Goodpasture's syndrome and rapidly progressive GN (antiglomerular basement membrane or anti-GBM antibodies); and membranoproliferative GN. A renal biopsy is necessary to differentiate among the various kinds (see page 35). Only APSGN is discussed in this section.

Types of glomerular lesions

Lesion	Characteristics
Diffuse	Relatively uniform involvement of most or all glomeruli; most common form of glomerulonephritis
Focal	Changes in only some glomeruli while others are normal
Segmental-local	Changes in one part of the glomerulus with other parts unaffected
Mesangial	Deposits of immunoglobulins in the mesangial matrix
Membranous	Thickening of the glomerular capillary wall
Proliferative	An increase in the number of glomerular cells
Sclerotic	Glomerular scarring from previous glomerular injury
Crescentic	The accumulation of proliferating cells within Bowman's space making the appearance of a crescent

(From McCance.)[16]

DIAGNOSTIC STUDIES AND FINDINGS

Diagnostic test	Findings
Laboratory tests	
Routine urinalysis	Hematuria: >0-5 RBCs per high power field
	Proteinuria: >30-150 mg/24 hr
	Color change: red, red-brown
	Sediment: RBC casts
Serum albumin	<3.5-5 g/dl
Serum lipid	>400-800 mg/dl
Serum creatinine	>1.2 mg/dl (men); 1.1 mg/dl (women)
Blood urea nitrogen (BUN)	>5-20 mg/dl
Hemoglobin (Hgb)/hematocrit (Hct)	Hgb: <15.5 ± 1.1 g (men); 13.7 ± 1 g (women); Hct: <46 ± 3.1% (men); 40.9 ± 3% (women)
*Complement (C3)	<400-800 µg/ml
*Circulating immune complex	>25 µg/ml aggregated human gamma globulin
*Cryoglobulins	Present
*Antistreptolysin 0	>25 Todd units
Creatinine clearance	<85-125 ml/min/1.73 mm^3 (men); <75-115 ml/min/1.73 mm^3 (women)
Culture of throat or skin lesion	Streptococcal organism may be present early in course of disease
Kidney-ureter-bladder (KUB) x-ray	Kidneys normal size, or slight bilateral enlargement
Renal biopsy	Diffuse endocapillary proliferation with many polymorphs in glomerular tuft; immunofluorescence reveals deposits of IgG, IgM, and C3

*Altered early in the course of the disease.

MEDICAL MANAGEMENT

GENERAL MANAGEMENT

The goals of treatment are to control edema, preserve renal perfusion, treat hypertension while avoiding postural hypotension, and treat any intercurrent infection.

Hemodialysis, peritoneal dialysis, or continuous arteriovenous hemofiltration (see pages 134 to 157).

Limit sodium intake to 500-1,000 mg/day.

Limit fluids to 500 ml plus amount equal to volume of urine for previous 24 hr.

Limit potassium intake (if hyperkalemia) to 1,500 mg/day.

Limit protein intake (if uremic) to 60 g/day.

Provide 2,500-3,500 calories/day.

Prescribe bed rest during acute phase of illness.

DRUG THERAPY

Antihypertensives: Clonidine (Catapres), diazoxide (Hyperstat IV), hydralazine (Apresoline), methyldopa (Aldomet), prazosin (Minipress), propranolol (Inderal).

Diuretics: Furosemide (Lasix), hydrochlorothiazide (Hydrodiuril).

Potassium-lowering agents: Sodium polystyrene sulfonate (Kayexalate), calcium gluconate, sodium bicarbonate, 50% glucose and regular insulin.

Antacids: Aluminum compounds to increase gastric pH and bind phosphate.

H$_2$ blockers: Cimetidine (Tagamet), ranitidine (Zantac).

Other agents as dictated by complications: Cardiac glycosides for congestive heart failure, antiinfectives if infection is still present, anticonvulsants.

1　ASSESS

ASSESSMENT	OBSERVATIONS
General complaints	Headache; low back pain; malaise; nausea; vomiting; fever; chills
Urine output	Decreased volume; dark brown or rust color
Cardiovascular system	Hypertension; edema

2　DIAGNOSE

NURSING DIAGNOSIS	SUBJECTIVE FINDINGS	OBJECTIVE FINDINGS
Altered renal tissue perfusion related to immunologic injury to kidney	Reports headache, low back pain	Vomiting; fever; chills; elevated blood pressure; oliguria
Fluid volume excess related to altered renal function	May report shortness of breath	Decreased urine output; edema; weight gain; jugular venous distention
Potential for altered nutrition: less than body requirements related to proteinuria	May complain of tiredness	Proteinuria, decreased serum albumin
Potential for infection related to altered immune state	None	Signs of infection in body excretions, secretions, exudates; fever, chills, positive cultures in blood, sputum, or urine

3　PLAN

Patient goals

1. The patient will demonstrate normal renal function.
2. The patient will demonstrate balance between fluid intake and output.
3. The patient's nutritional intake will be adequate for body's requirements.
4. The patient will be free of infection.
5. The patient will be knowledgeable about acute post-streptococcal glomerulonephritis and the treatment regimen.

4 IMPLEMENT

NURSING DIAGNOSIS	NURSING INTERVENTIONS	RATIONALE
Altered renal tissue perfusion related to immunologic injury to kidneys	Assess blood pressure q 6-8 hr, 24-hr intake and output, and edema; monitor laboratory data: serum potassium, serum creatinine, BUN, Hgb, Hct, carbon dioxide, serum phosphate, and urinalysis.	Acute renal failure may develop with azotemia, anemia, hyperkalemia, hyperphosphatemia, acidosis, and seizures.
	Administer antihypertensive agents as ordered; administer agents to lower potassium if needed; administer antacids used as phosphate-binding agents if ordered; administer anticonvulsant agents if ordered.	To control uremic symptoms and cardiovascular complications.
Fluid volume excess related to altered renal function	Assess for peripheral edema; weigh daily; measure blood pressure, pulse, and respirations q 6-8 h; measure 24-h intake and output.	To determine the extent of fluid retention.
	If volume excess is severe, assess pulmonary capillary wedge pressure and central venous pressure, jugular venous distention, breath sounds, and respiratory rate.	To assess cardiac function and pulmonary status.
	Limit sodium and fluid intake.	To limit fluid retention.
	Administer diuretic agents as ordered.	To mobilize retained fluids.
	Administer cardiac glycosides if ordered.	To prevent congestive heart failure.
Potential for altered nutrition: less than body requirements related to proteinuria	Assess for weight loss. Monitor food intake; monitor for anorexia, nausea, and vomiting; offer small, frequent feedings. Try to encourage protein intake of .75-1 g/kg body weight/day plus amount lost in 24-hr urine output.	Excessive protein losses may occur. To ensure adequate calorie intake and thus prevent metabolism of tissue proteins for energy.
	Limit protein and potassium if necessary (uremia).	To decrease excretory load on the kidneys and possible accumulation of potassium and hydrogen ions.
Potential for infection related to altered immune state	Assess for urinary tract infection; monitor temperature; monitor WBC. Avoid exposure to individuals with infections.	GN patients are susceptible to urinary tract infection because of their altered immune status.
	Administer antiinfective agents if ordered.	A streptococcal infection may still be present.
Knowledge deficit	See Patient Teaching.	

5 EVALUATE

PATIENT OUTCOME	DATA INDICATING THAT OUTCOME IS REACHED
Patient has normal renal function.	Renal function tests are within normal limits.
Patient's fluid intake balances output.	Urine output balances with intake; urine is clear; edema is gone; blood pressure is in normal range; weight is stable.
Patient's nutritional intake is adequate.	Proteinuria has resolved; serum albumin and lipid levels are normal.
Patient is free of infection.	No signs or symptoms of infection are noted.
Patient is knowledgeable about APSGN.	Patient can describe the signs, symptoms, and course of the disease; her level of renal function and possible problems; and the medical regimen prescribed.

PATIENT TEACHING

1. Explain APSGN, its signs, and symptoms, and the course of the disease.
2. Explain the medical regimen, if any, for discharge.
3. Explain follow-up care: monitoring of blood pressure and urinalysis (hematuria and proteinuria).

Interstitial Nephritis

Interstitial nephritis (IN) is an acute, often drug-induced renal disease that involves inflammatory damage to interstitial tissue.

Damage to interstitial tissue is the second most common cause (after glomerular disease) of chronic renal failure. Causes of IN include infection (e.g., streptococcal) and drug use (antibiotics such as methicillin and ampicillin, sulfonamides, phenindione, and phenytoin). Such drugs may cause dose-related toxic reactions or non-dose-related allergic reactions.

Interstitial nephritis also may arise from idiopathic causes. Early detection of drug reactions, infections, and urinary tract obstruction is useful. It is important to be alert to the possibility that some patients may abuse over-the-counter analgesics, especially those containing acetaminophen (see box).

PATHOPHYSIOLOGY

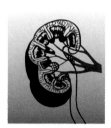

Acute inflammation of the interstitium may cause scarring and a rapid decline in renal function. As many as 10% to 15% of the cases of acute renal failure may be associated with acute interstitial nephritis.[14] The inflammatory process is usually diffuse and accompanied by interstitial edema. An immune response appears to cause acute IN that may involve deposition both of immune complexes and antitubular basement membrane antibodies.

Chronic IN results in a shrunken kidney with an irregular outline, caused by scarring and tissue destruction. It follows a slowly progressive course with few clinical manifestations. Changes in renal hormone activity may occur, and the production of renin, erythropoietin, and vitamin D may decline. The ability to concentrate urine also decreases. Common causes of chronic IN are anatomic abnormalities (e.g., obstruction in the urinary tract), analgesic use, hyperuricemia, and nephrosclerosis.

COMPLICATIONS

Renal failure

DIAGNOSTIC STUDIES AND FINDINGS

Diagnostic test	Findings
Laboratory tests	
White blood cell count	Eosinophilia
Urinalysis	Eosinophilic casts; hematuria; dilute urine (low specific gravity)
Intravenous urogram	Normal or slightly enlarged kidneys; immediate, dense nephrogram; with chronic interstitial nephritis: decreased size, irregular cortex, calyceal distortion
Renal biopsy	Differentiates acute tubular necrosis from acute interstitial nephritis

MEDICAL MANAGEMENT

GENERAL MANAGEMENT

The cause of IN can be removed by treating infection, discontinuing the drugs associated with the condition, and relieving obstruction. Renal function may gradually improve. Chronic IN requires monitoring as renal function decreases. Changes in the function of the glomeruli and tubules occur as the interstitial inflammation and scarring progress (see "Chronic Renal Failure," page 49).

DRUG THERAPY

Antiinfective agents: If needed.

SURGERY

Surgery may be performed to relieve any obstruction.

---

1 ASSESS

ASSESSMENT	OBSERVATIONS
Urinary tract	Polyuria; nocturia
Skin	May have an allergic skin rash

2 DIAGNOSE

NURSING DIAGNOSIS	SUBJECTIVE FINDINGS	OBJECTIVE FINDINGS
Altered renal tissue perfusion related to damaged interstitial tissue	Reports headache; low back pain	Nocturia; elevated blood pressure; altered mental status
Potential fluid volume deficit related to inability to concentrate urine or **potential for excess** related to acute renal failure associated with oliguria or anuria	None	Polyuria; weight loss Oliguria; weight gain; edema
Potential for infection related to damaged interstitium	None	Fever; chills

➜ ❯ ❯

3 PLAN

Patient goals

1. The patient will demonstrate normal renal function.
2. The patient will demonstrate normal fluid balance relationships.

3. The patient will be free of infection.
4. The patient will be knowledgeable about interstitial nephritis, its cause and treatment, and the implications for the future.

4 IMPLEMENT

NURSING DIAGNOSIS	NURSING INTERVENTIONS	RATIONALE
Altered renal tissue perfusion related to damaged interstitial tissue	Assess blood pressure q 6-8 h, 24-h intake and output, and edema; monitor laboratory data: Hgb/Hct; serum creatinine; BUN; serum potassium, phosphate, carbon dioxide. Urinalysis: specific gravity; monitor mental status.	Nonoliguric renal failure may develop with hypertension, azotemia, anemia, increased serum potassium and phosphate, and acidosis.
	Administer antihypertensive agents, agents to reduce serum potassium, and agents to reduce phosphate absorption as ordered; monitor response.	To control complications of uremia; and to determine effectiveness of drug, dosage, and timing.
Potential fluid volume deficit related to inability to concentrate urine or **potential for excess** related to acute renal failure associated with oliguria or anuria	Assess for dehydration; weigh daily; measure blood pressure, pulse, and respirations q 6-8 hr; measure 24-h intake and output.	To check for inability to concentrate urine and determine extent of fluid loss.
	Administer fluids as ordered; monitor response.	To prevent dehydration and further decrease in renal blood flow.
	Monitor for edema and listen to breath sounds; if fluid excess is severe, monitor central venous pressure and pulmonary capillary wedge pressure.	To identify hypervolemia.
Potential for infection related to damaged interstitium	Assess for signs and symptoms of urinary tract infection; administer antiinfective agents if ordered; monitor response to drug.	Renal failure alters immune response; monitoring determines effectiveness of drug, dosage, and timing.
Knowledge deficit	See Patient Teaching.	

5 EVALUATE

PATIENT OUTCOME	DATA INDICATING THAT OUTCOME IS REACHED
Renal function has returned.	Fluid and electrolyte balances are within normal limits; serum creatinine and BUN are normal.
Patient's fluid intake balances output.	Urine output equals intake; polyuria ceases; blood pressure is normal; weight is stable.
Patient is free of infection.	No signs or symptoms of infection are noted.
Patient is knowledgeable about interstitial nephritis.	Patient and family can describe the nature and extent of interstitial nephritis, the need for follow-up, and the implications for the future.

PATIENT TEACHING

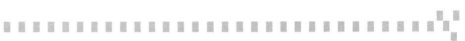

1. Explain the nature of interstitial nephritis and the cause in the individual patient.
2. Explain the patient's level of renal function.
3. Explain the need for periodic medical evaluation with tests of renal function.
4. Explain the likelihood of dialysis or transplantation in the future.

CHAPTER 7

Renovascular Diseases

Diabetic Nephropathy

Diabetic nephropathy (DN) is the renal manifestation of diabetes mellitus; it is glomerulosclerosis caused by lesions of the arterioles and glomeruli and associated with pyelonephritis and necrosis of the renal papillae.

Diabetic nephropathy, or diabetic glomerulosclerosis, is a very important complication of adult-onset diabetes mellitus and the most important complication leading to death in juvenile-onset diabetes. The changes are related to the duration of the diabetic state. All insulin-dependent diabetic patients can expect to develop DN. Once proteinuria occurs, the renal changes invariably progress (Figure 7-1). Patients with diabetic nephropathy have increased morbidity and mortality. Although the survival of diabetic patients treated with dialysis or transplantation has improved somewhat in recent years, the outcomes are not nearly as good as in nondiabetic patients. Diabetic patients have particular problems with atherosclerosis, coronary artery disease, peripheral vascular disease, retinopathy, and neurologic deficits. The likelihood of their successful rehabilitation is limited but has increased in recent years.

PATHOPHYSIOLOGY

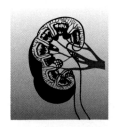
The glomeruli are affected by diffuse sclerosis and thickening of the basement membrane and mesangial areas. Nodular glomerulosclerosis may also occur. Both afferent and efferent arterioles are affected by thickened walls and hyaline deposits. The glomerular filtration rate decreases, and azotemia occurs. The diabetic patient may appear clinically uremic at GFR levels higher than

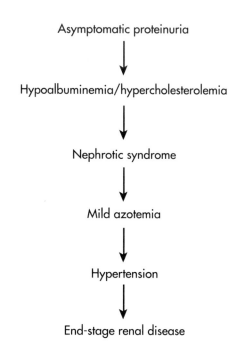

Asymptomatic proteinuria

↓

Hypoalbuminemia/hypercholesterolemia

↓

Nephrotic syndrome

↓

Mild azotemia

↓

Hypertension

↓

End-stage renal disease

FIGURE 7-1
Diabetic nephropathy—disease trajectory.

the nondiabetic patient. This may be related to the diabetic patient's systemic vascular changes.

Diabetic nephropathy may not manifest clinical symptoms for years after diabetes develops. Diabetic

> For a picture of diabetic nephropathy, see Color Plate 3 on page x.

individuals vary considerably in their susceptibility to renal failure, possibly because of genetic defects or vascular changes related to metabolism of carbohydrates, fat, and protein. Poor control of blood pressure and glucose levels appears to be important.

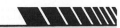
Acute renal failure	Urinary tract infection
Chronic renal failure	Pyelonephritis

MEDICAL MANAGEMENT

GENERAL MANAGEMENT

Some authorities believe that controlling blood pressure and fluctuations in blood sugar slows the deterioration of renal function. Others believe that diabetic nephropathy follows an inexorable downhill course.

Weight reduction is advocated. Protein is restricted early in the course of renal failure. Intermediate levels of renal failure require low-protein diets with drugs to lower cholesterol. Late in the course of renal failure, insulin requirements decrease but protein, carbohydrate, and fat intake must still be controlled.

Nutritional modifications are made to achieve or maintain adequate nutritional status and to reduce the work of diseased kidneys.

Protein: 0.6 g/kg body weight/day; glomerular filtration rate (GFR), 20-25 ml/min-90 g/day; GFR, 10-15 ml/min-50 g/day; GFR, 4-10 ml/min-40 g/day.

Sodium: 1,000-2,000 mg/day; specific amounts depend on weight, blood pressure, serum creatinine, and 24-hr sodium excretion.

Potassium: 1,500-2,000 mg/day; with normal urine output (at least 800 ml/day), no restriction is needed.

Calories: 35-55 kcal/kg body weight/day; calories from fat and carbohydrate are used; adequate calories must accompany protein intake to prevent use of protein for energy and weight loss; control of protein intake takes priority in nutritional management; calories from fat and carbohydrates are increased.

Fluid intake should balance output: About 400-600 ml (about amount of insensible losses) plus amount equal to 24-hr urine volume; avoid dehydration and volume excess; specific amount is determined by patient's dry weight (weight at which, after dialysis, patient has normal volume relationship).

See "Hemodialysis" and "Peritoneal Dialysis" (pages 134 and 145); the underlying disease process cannot be corrected by dialysis; vascular complications of diabetes cause major problems in access to vascular system for hemodialysis.

DRUG THERAPY

Antihypertensives: To control blood pressure; angiotensin-converting enzyme inhibitors may be particularly useful for their effect on intraglomerular pressure through relaxation of afferent arterioles.

Diuretics: May be needed.

Antiinfective agents: Infection is frequently a complication of nephropathy and chronic renal failure; agents specific to the microorganism cultured should be used. NOTE: Agents whose route of excretion is primarily renal need to be used in smaller doses or at lengthened intervals, depending on the GFR; agents excreted by only the liver require no change; if partial excretion occurs via the kidneys, some adjustment is needed at lower GFRs.

Insulin: Requirements may decrease as renal degradation of the hormone decreases or may increase as resistance to insulin's effects increases.

For noninsulin-dependent diabetic patients, use oral agents metabolized in the liver: tolbutamide (Orinase), glipizide (Glucotrol).

SURGERY

See "Renal Transplantation" (page 157). Diabetic patients who have a renal transplant have more complications, poorer rehabilitation, and a lower survival rate than nondiabetic patients with a renal transplant; the underlying disease process cannot be corrected by transplantation of kidney alone. Pancreas transplantation is being used in conjuction with the kidney transplant.

DIAGNOSTIC STUDIES AND FINDINGS

Diagnostic test	Findings
Laboratory tests	
Blood chemistries	Increased serum creatinine and BUN; decreased albumin; increased cholesterol
Urinalysis	Proteinuria, pyuria, or bacteriuria
Creatinine clearance	Lowered values
Intravenous urogram	Kidneys may be normal size, swollen, or small and scarred (irregular cortical surface)
Renal biopsy	Diffuse or nodular thickening of glomerular basement membrane and mesangial regions

1 ASSESS

ASSESSMENT	OBSERVATIONS
Cardiovascular	Hypertension; postural hypotension; edema or dehydration
Gastrointestinal	Nausea
Renal	Oliguria or anuria or urinary retention

2 DIAGNOSE

NURSING DIAGNOSIS	SUBJECTIVE FINDINGS	OBJECTIVE FINDINGS
Altered renal tissue perfusion related to diffuse and nodular glomerulosclerosis	None	Early: proteinuria; hypercholesterolemia; hypoalbuminemia; decreased GFR; azotemia; hypertension Late: end-stage renal disease
Altered nutrition related to change in renal handling of glucose	Complains of nausea; anorexia	Hyperglycemia; glycosuria
Potential for fluid volume deficit related to osmotic diuresis	Complains of thirst	Oliguria; increased specific gravity of urine; weight loss; dehydration
Potential for infection related to susceptibility because of diabetes and chronic renal failure	None	Signs and symptoms of infection in bodily excretions, secretions, and exudates; chills and fever; positive cultures in sputum, blood, or urine

3 PLAN

Patient goals

1. The patient will demonstrate stable or slowed progression of alteration in renal tissue perfusion.
2. The patient will demonstrate an adequate nutritional status.
3. The patient will demonstrate normal fluid balance.
4. The patient will have no infection.
5. The patient will be knowledgeable about diabetic nephropathy, its causes and course, the medical follow-up required, and the future need for dialysis or transplantation.
6. See also Chronic Renal Failure, page 49.

4 IMPLEMENT

NURSING DIAGNOSIS	NURSING INTERVENTIONS	RATIONALE
Altered renal tissue perfusion related to diffuse and nodular glomerulosclerosis	Assess vital signs, intake and output, and weight as needed; monitor laboratory values: serum glucose, BUN, serum creatinine.	Reflect status of diabetes and renal function.
	Administer medications as ordered with care.	Dosages are given in smaller amounts or at lengthened intervals.
	Determine insulin dose by serum glucose level.	Urine glucose level does not accurately reflect serum glucose level because of altered renal handling of glucose.
	Avoid nephrotoxic drugs.	Kidneys are less able to excrete drugs they normally handle.
	Monitor response to drugs.	To determine effectiveness of drug, dosage, and timing and identify adverse reactions.
Altered nutrition related to changes in renal handling of glucose	Assess food intake and dry weight; monitor laboratory data: serum glucose, urinary glucose; encourage food intake as ordered.	To assure adequate intake within limits prescribed.
Potential for fluid deficit related to osmotic diuresis	Assess neck veins, capillary refill, oral mucous membranes, and skin turgor q 4-6 h; monitor weight daily, also 24-h intake and output; assess blood pressure, pulse, and respirations q 6-8 h; assess central venous pressure and pulmonary artery wedge pressure q 6-8 h.	To identify changes in fluid status.
	Monitor laboratory data: serum glucose, serum sodium, potassium, chloride, and bicarbonate.	To identify electrolytes lost with fluid losses.

→ > > >

NURSING DIAGNOSIS	NURSING INTERVENTIONS	RATIONALE
Potential for infection related to increased susceptibility with diabetes and chronic renal failure	Assess for signs and symptoms of infection in secretions, excretions, and exudates; assess for fever; monitor temperature q 4-6 h; monitor laboratory data: WBC.	To detect infection early.
	Ensure aseptic technique for any invasive procedure or wound care.	To decrease chances of infection.
Knowledge deficit	See Patient Teaching. See also Chronic Renal Failure, page 49.	

5 EVALUATE

PATIENT OUTCOME	DATA INDICATING THAT OUTCOME IS REACHED
Renal tissue perfusion is adequate.	Renal function test results are normal or stable.
Fluid balance is within normal limits.	Urinary output balances input.
Nutritional status is adequate.	Food and fluid restrictions are appropriate to level of renal function and diabetic needs.
No infection is present.	No signs or symptoms of infection are noted.
Patient and family are knowledgeable about diabetic nephropathy.	Patient and family can explain diabetic nephropathy, its causes, manifestations, and treatment; medical follow-up; and the potential for dialysis or transplantation in the future.

PATIENT TEACHING

1. Explain the nature of diabetic nephropathy and chronic renal failure.
2. Explain the medical regimen and its rationale, including diet (restricted protein, sodium, and potassium), restricted fluid intake, and medications (purpose, dosage, interval, and adverse reactions).
3. Teach the patient self-observational skills (temperature, pulse, respirations, blood pressure, intake and output, and weight) and record keeping.
4. Explain avoidance of infection.
5. Explain personal hygiene, rest, and exercise.
6. Explain when to call the physician.
7. Explain the plan for medical follow-up.
8. Explain renal dialysis and transplantation.

Nephrosclerosis

Severe hypertension can cause renal function to deteriorate. **Nephrosclerosis** is the damage to the renal arteries, arterioles, and glomeruli caused by prolonged elevated blood pressure.

Renal parenchymal disease is a major consequence of prolonged elevated blood pressure. Important factors in the development of such problems are the age at which hypertension occurs, its severity, and the presence of risk factors (e.g., race, family history of hypertension or cardiovascular disease, obesity, diabetes mellitus, smoking, lack of exercise). Many people develop arteriosclerosis and atherosclerosis as they age; such changes are accelerated with hypertension.

PATHOPHYSIOLOGY

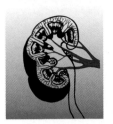

A slow, variable progression of vascular changes can occur over the years. The process includes spasm, thickening, hypertrophy, and hyaline degeneration of the renal arterial system. In malignant hypertension, renal changes are rapid and include fibrinoid necrosis. The damaged kidney decreases or stops production of substances that lower blood pressure.

COMPLICATIONS

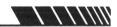

Acute renal failure
Chronic renal failure

For a picture of nephrosclerosis, see Color Plate 4, page x.

MEDICAL MANAGEMENT

The goals of therapy include aggressively controlling blood pressure to slow renal deterioration, delaying end-stage renal disease by conservative management, and beginning dialysis or performing a renal transplant at the appropriate point in the course of the disease. Drug dosages and intervals must be modified when the kidneys are involved in the drug's excretion. Rates of excretion and metabolism and sensitivity to drugs may be altered.

GENERAL MANAGEMENT

Bed rest, sodium restriction, and antihypertensive drugs are basic.
Fluid intake to balance output: about 400-600 ml (about the amount of insensible losses) plus amount equal to 24-hr urine volume; patient should avoid dehydration and volume excess.
Nutritional modifications to achieve or maintain adequate nutritional status and to reduce work of diseased kidney: Protein: 0.6 g/kg body weight/day; glomerular filtration rate (GFR) 20-25 ml/min-90 g/day; GFR 10-15 ml/min-50 g/day; GFR 4-10 ml/min-40 g/day.
Sodium: 1,000-2,000 mg/day; specific amounts depend on weight, blood pressure, serum creatinine, and 24-hr sodium excretion.
Potassium: 1,500-2,000 mg/day; with normal urine output (at least 800 ml/day), no restriction needed.
Calories: 35-55 kcal/kg body weight/day; calories from fat and carbohydrate used; adequate calories must accompany protein intake to prevent use of protein for energy and weight loss.
If chronic renal failure develops, dialysis by home or incenter hemodialysis, home or incenter intermittent peritoneal dialysis, or continuous ambulatory peritoneal dialysis (CAPD) may be needed; (see page 134.)

MEDICAL MANAGEMENT—cont'd

DRUG THERAPY

Single- or multiple-drug therapy is used in a stepwise progression as drug effects are monitored (see Figure 7-2).

Antihypertensives: Adrenergic blocking agents, vasodilators, angiotensin-converting enzyme blockers, and calcium slow channel blockers.

Diuretics: Thiazides, loop diuretics, and potassium-sparing diuretics.

Surgery: Renal transplantation may be an option in the future.

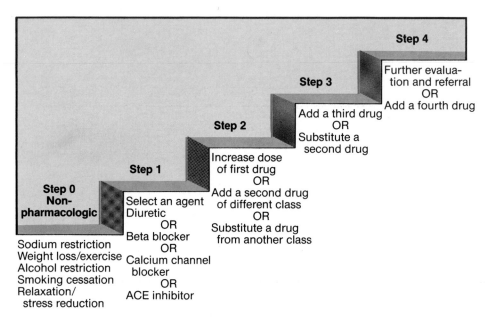

FIGURE 7-2
Stepped-care approach to treatment of high blood pressure.
(From Canobbio.[2])

DIAGNOSTIC STUDIES AND FINDINGS

Diagnostic test	Findings
Laboratory tests	
Urinalysis	Proteinuria; hematuria
Blood chemistries	BUN, serum creatinine above normal; serum potassium low; serum calcium elevated
Kidney-ureter-bladder (KUB) x-ray	Small kidneys, bilaterally
Intravenous urogram	Small kidneys, bilaterally
Electrocardiogram (ECG)	Left ventricular hypertrophy

1   ASSESS

ASSESSMENT	OBSERVATIONS
Cardiovascular	Elevated blood pressure; tachycardia; fourth heart sound, forceful point of maximum impulse
Optic fundi	Retinal blood vessel changes: narrowing, hemorrhages, and exudates
General complaints	Headache, dizziness, fatigue, palpitations, blurred vision

2   DIAGNOSE

NURSING DIAGNOSIS	SUBJECTIVE FINDINGS	OBJECTIVE FINDINGS
Altered renal tissue perfusion related to damage to nephrons by hypertension	None	Nocturia; proteinuria; hematuria

3   PLAN

Patient goals

1. The patient will demonstrate stable renal tissue perfusion.

2. The patient will be knowledgeable about nephrosclerosis, its causes and treatment, medical follow-up, and the potential need for dialysis and transplantation in the future.

4   IMPLEMENT

NURSING DIAGNOSIS	NURSING INTERVENTIONS	RATIONALE
Altered renal tissue perfusion related to damage to nephrons by hypertension	Assess standing and lying blood pressures and pulse q 4-6 h; record weight daily; calculate 24-h intake and output.	To identify increased peripheral vascular resistance, postural hypotension, and fluid retention.
	Administer medications as ordered.	Dosages may be reduced and time intervals lengthened for drugs excreted by kidneys.
	Observe response to drugs.	To determine effectiveness of drug, dosage, and timing and to identify adverse reactions.
	Monitor laboratory data: serum potassium, calcium, uric acid, bicarbonate, pH, and glucose.	These substances may be altered when taking diuretics and in chronic renal failure.

→ › ›

NURSING DIAGNOSIS	NURSING INTERVENTIONS	RATIONALE
	Follow ECG changes.	ECG changes associated with hyperkalemia are peaked T wave, prolonged PR interval, widened QRS complex, and cardiac standstill.
	Watch for Kussmaul breathing and Chvostek's or Trousseau's signs.	To identify acidosis and hypocalcemia.
Knowledge deficit	See Patient Teaching.	

5   EVALUATE

PATIENT OUTCOME	DATA INDICATING THAT OUTCOME IS REACHED
Renal tissue perfusion is stable.	Renal function findings do not worsen.
Patient and family are knowledgeable about nephrosclerosis.	Patient and family can describe nephrosclerosis, the medical plan of care, and future options for renal dialysis or transplantation.

PATIENT TEACHING

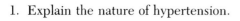

1. Explain the nature of hypertension.

2. Explain the nature of chronic renal failure. (See page 185.)

Renal Artery Occlusion or Stenosis and Renal Vein Thrombosis

Renal artery occlusion is a sudden, complete blockage of the renal artery or a branch of it. **Stenosis** is a narrowing of the artery. The renal vein or a branch of it can be blocked by an **embolus** or **thrombus.**

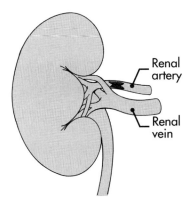

Renal
artery

Renal
vein

Renal artery occlusion

Renal artery problems frequently are associated with atherosclerosis (in older patients) and fibromuscular hyperplasia. Renal vein thrombosis is most frequently associated with nephrotic syndrome (NS). It also may accompany an aortic aneurysm, a hematoma, trauma, or a neoplasm that compresses the renal vein.

PATHOPHYSIOLOGY

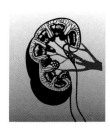

In renal artery occlusion, complete cessation of arterial blood flow causes an infarct, with coagulation necrosis in the kidney. If the person has a single kidney, acute oliguric renal failure ensues. Occlusion is most frequently the result of an embolism caused by mitral valve stenosis, subacute bacterial endocarditis, and mural thrombi after a myocardial infarction.

Severe stenosis caused by atherosclerosis leads to ischemic atrophy and fibrosis. Decreased pressure in the arterioles stimulates the juxtaglomerular apparatus to increase renin secretion and can lead to renovascular hypertension.

A sudden, complete occlusion of the renal vein causes an infarct; the kidney swells, pressing against the capsule. If an occlusion evolves slowly, however, collateral venous circulation may develop, resulting in less impairment of renal function. Renal vein thrombosis may be associated with dehydration, sepsis, or hypercoagulability states.

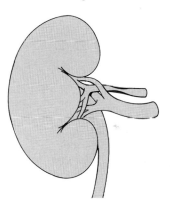

Renal artery stenosis

For pictures of renal artery thrombosis and renal artery embolism, see Color Plates 5 and 6, pages x and xi.

COMPLICATIONS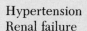

Hypertension
Renal failure

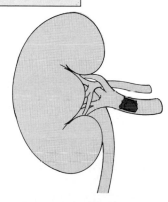

Renal vein thrombosis

DIAGNOSTIC STUDIES AND FINDINGS

Diagnostic tests	Findings		
	Renal artery occlusion	**Renal artery stenosis**	**Renal vein thrombosis**
Intravenous urogram	Affected kidney is smaller, calyces are smaller, nephrogram phase is delayed		Unilateral change in kidney function when radiopaque dye is injected: enlargement, poorly visualized
Renal arteriogram	Absence of function in all or part of the kidney as it filters radiopaque dye		
Renal venogram			Demonstrable clot
Laboratory tests			
Urine	Microscopic hematuria		Gross hematuria; proteinuria; foamy, deep yellow color
Complete blood count	Leukocytosis		Signs of nephrotic syndrome
Blood chemistries	Increased lactic dehydrogenase (LDH)		
Plasma renin activity		Increased level in renal vein	

MEDICAL MANAGEMENT

GENERAL MANAGEMENT

A conservative approach is used in the treatment of these renal disorders. Patients usually have serious cardiac disease. Pain relief is a major focus in occlusion; with stenosis, blood pressure must be controlled; and with renal vein thrombosis, preventing pulmonary emboli is vital. The underlying cause of NS should be treated if possible (see "Nephrotic Syndrome"), and other disease states must be treated.
Monitor contralateral kidney function. Stabilize cardiac function.
Dialysis may be needed with any of these conditions.

DRUG THERAPY

Antihypertensives: In renal artery stenosis. (Angiotensin converting enzyme inhibitors)

Anticoagulants: Heparin in renal artery occlusion and renal vein thrombosis.

Thrombolytics: May or may not be helpful in renal artery occlusion. (Streptokinase)

Analgesics: Both renal artery occlusion and stenosis are painful conditions (Morphine, Meperidine).

SURGERY

Embolectomies are not usually performed for renal artery occlusion; renal damage usually has occurred by time diagnosis is made.
Selected patients with renal artery stenosis may have surgical correction; percutaneous transluminal angioplasty may be used.
If a thrombus begins in the aorta and extends into the renal artery, percutaneous transluminal angioplasty is less successful than if only renal artery is involved.
Aortorenal bypass; autogenous vascular graft.
A nephrectomy may be needed in renal artery stenosis for renovascular hypertension that does not respond to drug therapy (see page 165).

1 ASSESS

ASSESSMENT	OBSERVATIONS		
	RENAL ARTERY OCCLUSION	RENAL ARTERY STENOSIS	RENAL VEIN THROMBOSIS
Cardiovascular		Hypertension; abdominal bruits	
General	Pain in flank or upper abdomen; few signs if infarct is small		Flank pain

2 DIAGNOSE

NURSING DIAGNOSIS	SUBJECTIVE FINDINGS	OBJECTIVE FINDINGS
Altered renal tissue perfusion related to altered arterial or venous flow	None	Oliguria; hypertension
Pain related to impeded blood flow	Complains of flank or upper abdominal pain	Guarding behavior

3 PLAN

Patient goals
1. The patient will demonstrate improved renal tissue perfusion.
2. The patient will be free of pain.
3. The patient will be knowledgeable about the renal vascular condition, its causes, and the treatment regimen.

4 IMPLEMENT

NURSING DIAGNOSIS	NURSING INTERVENTIONS	RATIONALE
Altered renal tissue perfusion related to altered arterial or venous flow	Assess vital signs q 4-6 h; assess weight daily.	To determine systemic effects of renal problem.
	Assess neck veins, central venous pressure, and pulmonary capillary wedge pressure if appropriate; monitor blood pressure both lying and standing q 4 h; monitor intake and output daily; monitor laboratory data: urine protein, BUN, serum creatinine, and clotting times.	To determine effect on cardiovascular and renal function.

→ 〉 〉

NURSING DIAGNOSIS	NURSING INTERVENTIONS	RATIONALE
	Give antihypertensive and anticoagulant agents as ordered; observe response to drugs.	To determine effectiveness of drug and dosage and observe for adverse and toxic side effects.
Pain related to altered arterial or venous flow	Assess pattern of pain, and determine need for analgesia; administer analgesics as ordered, and observe response to drug given.	Sudden increase may mean extention of problem. To promote comfort; to determine the effectiveness of drug, dosage, and timing and identify adverse reactions.
Knowledge deficit	See Patient Teaching.	

5 EVALUATE

PATIENT OUTCOME	DATA INDICATING THAT OUTCOME IS REACHED
Some function has returned after renal artery occlusion.	Patient's renal function tests show improvement.
Medical therapy or surgery has helped with renal artery stenosis.	Hypertension has been relieved or is under control.
Renal function has returned completely or is now impaired in renal vein thrombosis.	Renal function test results are normal or reflect degrees of impairment.

PATIENT TEACHING

1. Explain the nature of renal artery occlusion, renal artery stenosis, or renal vein thrombosis.

2. Explain the treatment regimen and its rationale.
3. Explain the follow-up medical care required.

CHAPTER 8

Metabolic Disorders

Renal Calculi

Renal calculi are stones formed in the kidneys, primarily in the pelvis (Figure 8-1). Stones may resemble gravel or may be formed in the shape of the pelvis (staghorn calculus).

Calculi that pass spontaneously without discomfort present no serious health threat. However, many calculi found in the urinary tract are extremely painful and can cause obstruction and infection. Urinary calculi occur more frequently in men than in women, and some geographic areas, such as the southeastern United States, have a particularly high incidence. The peak incidence of calculus formation is in the third to fifth decades of life.

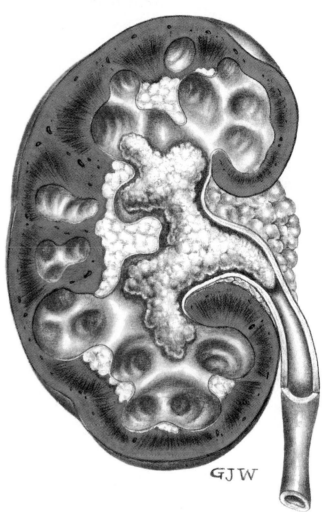

GJW

Staghorn calculus

For a picture of a staghorn calculus, see Color Plate 7, page xi.

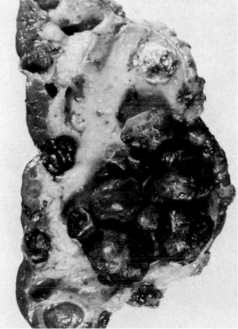

FIGURE 8-1
Hydronephrosis with renal stones in renal pelvis and calyces. (From Kissane.[13])

Long-term ingestion of calcium carbonate, vitamin D, antacids, megadoses of vitamin C, acetazolamide, probenecid, or triamterene can lead to stone formation. The risk can be increased by anatomic abnormalities (medullary sponge kidney), biochemical influences (cystinuria), or environmental factors (diet and fluid intake patterns, climate, occupation).

PATHOPHYSIOLOGY

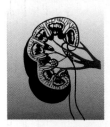

The formation of a stone is a physiochemical process involving a nidus of crystals or organic material around which the stone components form. The pH, temperature, ionic strength, and concentration of the urine affect the solubility of the stone-forming substances. Supersaturation of poorly soluble substances, absence of crystalline inhibitors, and sources of seed crystals contribute to calculus formation.

The primary components of renal calculi are calcium salts (carbonate and oxalate), uric acid, cystine, and struvite (magnesium ammonium phosphate). The stones most frequently contain calcium or uric acid.

Hypercalciuria with or without hypercalcemia may be caused by hyperparathyroidism or osteoporosis or may be idiopathic. Calcium and phosphate are more soluble when pH is low. Bacterial infection by urea-splitting organisms causes the urine to become alkaline. Stones composed of struvite are called infection stones.

Hyperuricemia occurs with idiopathic gout, renal failure, blood dyscrasias, and use of thiazide diuretics and alkylating agents. Uric acid is less soluble in high concentrations, low urine volume, and with low urine pH.

COMPLICATIONS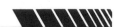

Infection
Obstruction

DIAGNOSTIC STUDIES AND FINDINGS

Diagnostic test	Findings
Kidney-ureter-bladder (KUB) x-ray	Radiopaque stone
Renal ultrasound	Stones identified
Intravenous urogram	Filling defects; ureteral dilation; hydronephrosis
Analysis of stones	Constituents such as cystine, calcium, oxalate, uric acid

MEDICAL MANAGEMENT

GENERAL MANAGEMENT

The goals of medical care are to remove calculi, relieve the effects of the calculi (pain and infection), resolve any causative factors (obstruction, infection, and metabolic abnormalities), and prevent future calculus growth. Accomplishing these goals should prevent permanent damage to the kidneys and recurrence of calculi.

Diet: Modifications may be required, depending on stone type.
Low-calcium diets (<400 mg/day) and extra-high fluid intake (3,500-4,000 ml/day) are helpful but difficult to maintain; patients should avoid dehydration by drinking water rather than fluids that may be high in unwanted substances (such as tea with its high oxalate content); increased fluid intake should be spread out evenly over the 24-hr period, including once during the night; low-purine diets may help decrease uric acid output; foods extremely high in purines (>150 mg/100 g) are limited; oxalate intake is usually limited to less than 50 mg/day on low-oxylate diets.

DRUG THERAPY

Analgesics: Meperidine (Demerol), morphine sulfate, codeine sulfate.
Diuretics: Hydrochlorothiazide (Hydrodiuril) to decrease idiopathic urinary calcium excretion.
Alkalinizing agents: To raise urinary pH: sodium bicarbonate.
Purine metabolism inhibitor: Allopurinol (Zyloprim).
For cystine stones: Penicillamine (combines with cystine to form a soluble product removed by the kidneys).
Antibiotics: For infection, if present.

MEDICAL MANAGEMENT—cont'd

SURGERY

Procedures used may include pyelolithotomy, nephrolithotomy, ureterolithotomy, cystoscopy-basket extraction of calculi, and percutaneous fragmentation and extraction through a nephroscope; surgical intervention is a last resort with struvite stones because recurrence is so common (see page 165).

Additional procedures: Extracorporeal shock-wave lithotripsy, percutaneous lithotripsy (see page 174).

1 ASSESS

ASSESSMENT	OBSERVATIONS
General	Fever (with urinary tract infection); pain associated with renal colic; nausea; vomiting
Urination	Irritative voiding behaviors: dysuria, urgency, and urge incontinence

2 DIAGNOSE

NURSING DIAGNOSIS	SUBJECTIVE FINDINGS	OBJECTIVE FINDINGS
Pain related to presence of renal calculus	Complains of pain in flank or costovertebral angle radiating to groin, labia, or testicle; complains of nausea	Guarding behavior; vomiting
Altered nutrition: more than body requirements related to altered metabolism of calcium, purine, or oxylate	None	Hypercalcemia or hypocalcemia; hypercalciuria; cystinuria; hyperuricemia; elevated uric acid in urine
Potential for infection related to presence of calculi	Complains of irritative voiding behaviors	Bacteriuria; pyuria; WBC casts; hematuria; elevated WBC

3 PLAN

Patient goals

1. The patient will be free of pain.
2. The patient will maintain an adequate fluid intake and limit intake of substances associated with calculus formation.
3. The patient will be free of signs and symptoms of urinary tract infection.
4. The patient will be knowledgeable about renal calculi and ways to prevent their recurrence.

→ > >

4 IMPLEMENT

NURSING DIAGNOSIS	NURSING INTERVENTIONS	RATIONALE
Pain related to presence of calculus	Note pattern of pain, and assess need for analgesia.	Intensified pain may indicate impaction of calculus or obstruction of urine flow; sudden relief of pain may indicate stone has passed through a narrow junction (ureteropelvic or ureterovesicle); movement of calculus may be associated with colicky pain.
	Administer analgesic agents as ordered; monitor response to drugs.	To relieve pain and to determine effectiveness of drug, amount, and timing.
	Apply external heat to painful flank.	To relieve discomfort.
	Assist with walking as ordered.	To help passage of stone.
Altered nutrition: more than body requirements related to altered metabolism of calcium, purine, or oxylate	For calcium stones, lower calcium intake (e.g., dairy products); for uric acid stones, decrease purine intake (e.g., organ meats, meat extracts, shrimp, and dried beans); lower intake of foods containing oxylate (e.g., tea, chocolate, nuts, and spinach).	To prevent formation of renal calculi.
	Avoid dehydration by encouraging high-normal fluid intake while avoiding unwanted substances.	To prevent high concentrations of unwanted substances in the urine.
Potential for infection related to presence of calculus	Assess for fever, chills, and irritative voiding symptoms; monitor laboratory data: WBC, bacteriuria; monitor temperature q 4 h.	To detect presence of infection.
	Encourage high-normal fluid intake over 24 h.	To help flush urinary tract to prevent urinary tract infection; may also facilitate passage of calculus.
Knowledge deficit	See Patient Teaching.	

5 EVALUATE

PATIENT OUTCOME	DATA INDICATING THAT OUTCOME IS REACHED
Pain is gone.	Patient reports being pain free.
No signs or symptoms of urinary tract infection are noted.	Temperature, urine, WBC are normal.

PATIENT OUTCOME	DATA INDICATING THAT OUTCOME IS REACHED
Fluid intake is adequate, and unwanted substances are avoided in the diet.	Fluid intake is high end of normal; diet restrictions are followed correctly.
Patient is knowledgeable about renal calculi.	Patient can explain factors that contribute to calculi and the signs and symptoms of recurrence.

PATIENT TEACHING

1. Explain the nature of renal calculi, their causes, and manifestations.
2. Explain medical management, including medications (purpose, dosage, interval, and side effects), diet (low calcium, purine, or oxylate), and fluid intake (amount, schedule, and kinds).
3. Explain medical follow-up to monitor the outcome of treatment.

Renal Tubular Acidosis

Renal tubular acidosis (RTA) occurs when the kidneys are unable to excrete an acid urine because of a defect in the tubules. Hyperchloremic acidosis ensues.

Both infants and adults may have tubular defects in acid handling. The causes of RTA may be hereditary or associated with cystinosis and hyperparathyroidism.

PATHOPHYSIOLOGY

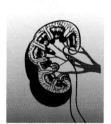

The tubular defect in RTA may be in the proximal tubule or the distal tubule. In the former case, the proximal tubule fails to conserve bicarbonate ions and the distal tubule, which is normal, cannot handle the increased bicarbonate load. Sodium and potassium are also lost, and hypokalemia and hypovolemia may result. In the latter case, the distal tubule cannot maintain the hydrogen ion gradient across the tubular cell and either fails to secrete hydrogen ions or permits back diffusion of the hydrogen ions secreted. The serum pH is lowered, the hydrogen-sodium exchange decreases, and the sodium-potassium exchange increases, with a resulting hypokalemia and hypovolemia.

The skeletal system becomes involved in buffering the acidosis; calcium carbonate is released, causing hypercalcemia and hypercalciuria. Renal function is otherwise normal. A third type of RTA involves defects in both parts of the tubule and a normal or elevated serum potassium. Renal calculi occur frequently in patients with distal RTA (see page 100).

COMPLICATIONS

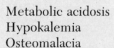

Metabolic acidosis
Hypokalemia
Osteomalacia
Renal calculi
Nephrocalcinosis

DIAGNOSTIC STUDIES AND FINDINGS

Diagnostic test	Findings
Laboratory tests	
Blood chemistries	Lowered serum pH and potassium; elevated serum chloride and calcium
Urinalysis	Urine pH >6 in distal RTA; 4.5-8 in proximal RTA with increased potassium level and hypercalciuria
Kidney-ureter-bladder (KUB) x-ray	Decreased kidney mass; renal calculi or intrarenal calcification

---

MEDICAL MANAGEMENT

GENERAL MANAGEMENT

There is no cure for renal tubular acidosis; therefore the major goal of therapy is to control the metabolic acidosis with moderate doses of bicarbonate.

DRUG THERAPY

Alkalinizing agents (for distal RTA): Sodium bicarbonate, sodium citrate and citric acid (Shohl's Solution), Polycitra. NOTE: The acidosis must be corrected slowly to avoid lowering the potassium level further.

Diuretics (for proximal RTA): Hydrochlorothiazide (Hydrodiuril) to decrease calcium excretion.

Potassium supplement (for proximal RTA): Potassium chloride.

---

1   ASSESS

ASSESSMENT	OBSERVATIONS
General	Weakness; lethargy; anorexia; bone pain

2   DIAGNOSE

NURSING DIAGNOSIS	SUBJECTIVE FINDINGS	OBJECTIVE FINDINGS
Potential for altered acid-base balance related to defect in renal tubule causing metabolic acidosis	None	Hyperchloremic metabolic acidosis; hypokalemia; hypercalciuria; alkaline urine

3 PLAN

Patient goals

1. The patient with proximal RTA will have a serum pH level in the low normal range.
2. The patient with distal RTA will have normal potassium, serum pH, and urinary calcium levels.
3. The patient will be knowledgeable about the causes, signs and symptoms, and treatment of renal tubular acidosis.

4 IMPLEMENT

NURSING DIAGNOSIS	NURSING INTERVENTIONS	RATIONALE
Potential for altered acid-base balance related to defect in renal tubule causing metabolic acidosis	Monitor laboratory values: serum hydrogen, bicarbonate, calcium, potassium, and pH; urinary pH and calcium.	To assess effectiveness of medical regimen.
	Administer medications as ordered.	To treat acidosis and prevent electrolyte losses.
Knowledge deficit	See Patient Teaching.	

5 EVALUATE

PATIENT OUTCOME	DATA INDICATING THAT OUTCOME IS REACHED
Acid-base imbalance has been corrected; potassium level is normal, and nephrocalcinosis and renal calculi have been prevented.	Urine pH is 4.5-8; urine calcium is 2-3 mg/kg/day; serum bicarbonate is 24-28 mEq/L; serum chloride is 97-107 mEq/L; serum potassium is 3.5-5 mEq/L; serum pH is 7.32-7.43. No renal calculi or calcifications are noted.
Patient and family are knowledgeable about RTA.	Patient and family can describe RTA and the medical management being instituted.

PATIENT TEACHING

1. Explain the nature of renal tubular acidosis.
2. Explain the treatment regimen: alkalinizing agent with dosage, interval, and side effects.
3. Teach the patient to check urine for pH and calcium.
4. Explain medical follow-up.

Nephrotic Syndrome

Nephrotic syndrome (NS) encompasses a group of symptoms: proteinuria (primarily albuminuria), hypoalbuminemia, generalized edema, hyperlipidemia, and lipiduria. NS occurs in both adults and children.

NS may occur in various conditions, such as glomerulonephritis, glomerular lesions associated with such systemic diseases and conditions as diabetes mellitus, infections, circulatory diseases, reactions to allergens and drugs, pregnancy, and renal transplantation. NS is frequently idiopathic in children. Long-term studies are under way to determine the usefulness of corticosteroids and cyclophosphamide in children and adults.

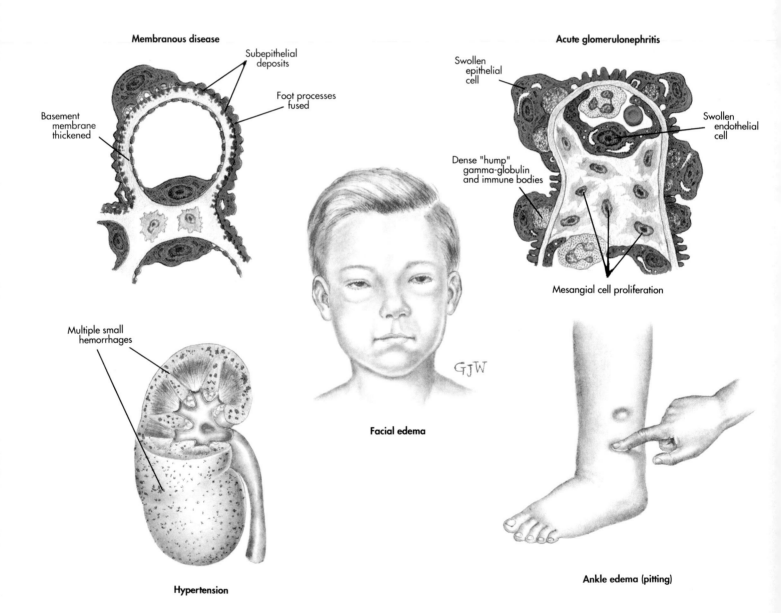

Membranous disease

Subepithelial deposits

Foot processes fused

Basement membrane thickened

Acute glomerulonephritis

Swollen epithelial cell

Dense "hump" gamma-globulin and immune bodies

Swollen endothelial cell

Mesangial cell proliferation

Multiple small hemorrhages

Facial edema

Hypertension

Ankle edema (pitting)

Table 8-1

CLINICAL MANIFESTATIONS OF NEPHROTIC SYNDROME

Manifestation	Contributing factors	Result
Proteinuria	Increased glomerular permeability, decreased proximal tubule reabsorption	Edema, increased susceptibility to infection from loss of immunoglobulins
Hypoalbuminemia	Increased urinary losses of protein	Edema
Edema	Hypoalbuminemia (decreased oncotic pressure, sodium and water retention, increased aldosterone and ADH secretion)	Soft, pitting, generalized edema
Hyperlipidemia	Decreased serum albumin; increased hepatic synthesis of very low-density lipoproteins; increased cholesterol, phospholipids, triglycerides	Increased atherogenesis
Lipiduria	Sloughing of tubular cells containing fat (oval fat bodies); free fat from hyperlipidemia	Fat droplets that may float in urine
Decreased vitamin D	The globulin, to which the active form of vitamin D is attached for transport, passing through glomerulus and lost in urine	Decreased absorption of calcium from gut

(From McCance.[16])

PATHOPHYSIOLOGY

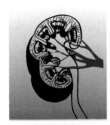

Nephrotic syndrome results from increased glomerular permeability. The albuminuria causes hypoalbuminemia, because the liver cannot replace the losses rapidly enough. The resulting drop in oncotic pressure permits water to escape from the vascular compartment. Adaptive responses to the contraction of fluid volume include increased secretion of antidiuretic hormone and aldosterone, which contributes to the problem of fluid retention. The liver is stimulated to increase the synthesis of many proteins and also production of lipoproteins, thereby causing the hyperlipidemia characteristic of NS (Table 8-1).

A renal biopsy in patients with NS may show either minimum or marked changes, including proliferation of endothelial cells (hypercellularity), changes in the epithelial cells (diffuse fusion of the foot processes), deposition of immunoglobulins and complexes along the capillary walls, tubular changes (fatty deposits and eosinophilic casts), and glomerular changes (epithelial crescents caused by irregular patches of sclerosis).

Most patients with NS who have minimum changes respond well to corticosteroid therapy. Patients with marked changes are usually unresponsive and progress to end-stage renal disease.

The decrease in plasma proteins may result in less binding proteins for drugs. The usual effect of a drug may occur with half the usual dose. The protein loss may also cause a decrease in vitamin D precursor, transferrin, triiodothyronine (T_3), and thyroid-binding globulin. Calcium may be required, but thyroid hormone usually is not. Iron may be needed if iron-deficiency anemia occurs.

COMPLICATIONS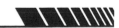

Infection	Thromboembolism
Atherosclerosis	Electrolyte imbalances

DIAGNOSTIC STUDIES AND FINDINGS

Diagnostic test	Findings
Laboratory tests	
Urine	Foamy, deeper in color; oval fat bodies; proteinuria that may be >3 g/day
Blood chemistry	Hypoalbuminemia: serum albumin <2.5 g/dl; hyperlipidemia: increased total serum cholesterol, phospholipids, triglycerides, low-density lipids, very-low-density lipids
Renal biopsy	To identify histologic features of lesion classified as:
	Minimum change—podocytes of epithelial cells appear to be fused together on electron microscopy
	Membranous change—predominantly thickening of the basement membrane and visible by light and electron microscopy
	Proliferative change—glomerular cells appear hypercellular
	Membranoproliferative change—both hypercellularity and basement membrane thickening are noted

MEDICAL MANAGEMENT

GENERAL MANAGEMENT

Protein intake is increased to replace urinary protein losses. If the glomerular filtration rate (GFR) is normal, adults may have 1.5-2 g/kg body weight. If the GFR is decreased, protein intake is lowered. Sodium intake is limited (500-1,000 mg/day) to control edema. Caloric intake must be sufficient to prevent muscle catabolism and provide energy. The amount varies with height, weight, age, sex, and daily activity. Adults need 35-45 kcal/kg ideal body weight/day. The help of a dietitian and the use of exchange lists make implementing these complex diets easier.

Changes in vascular volume are monitored carefully to prevent hypovolemic shock, as well as the hypokalemia and ototoxicity that can accompany diuretic use. Hospitalization is avoided unless the patient has severe generalized edema with ascites, significant hypertension, severe infection, hypovolemic shock, or a persistently low GFR. Bed rest is advised if complications are present. The level of proteinuria is monitored.

DRUG THERAPY

Immunosuppressive agents: Corticosteroids (prednisone); antineoplastic agents (i.e., cyclophosphamide [Cytoxan], azathioprine (Imuran), chlorambucil (Leukeran).

Plasma expander/blood component: Human albumin (Albuminate).

Diuretics: Furosemide (Lasix), hydrochlorothiazide (Hydrodiuril), spironolactone (Aldactone).

Protein diet supplements: Meritene, Citrotein.

NOTE: Immunosuppressive agents are used because they have been shown empirically to decrease or stop the proteinuria. Prednisone, the treatment of choice, is initially given as a single dose at breakfast and may be given later on alternate days. The other immunosuppressive agents are used if corticosteroids cannot be used. Diuretics are often used in conjunction with salt-poor albumin infusions to relieve massive edema. Thoracentesis or paracentesis may be needed if excess fluid accumulates in the chest or abdominal cavities. In minimum-disease NS, corticosteroids are started and the responses noted. Often proteinuria clears rapidly. Repeat treatment with corticosteroids is indicated for those who have a relapse after therapy is discontinued.

1 ASSESS

ASSESSMENT	OBSERVATIONS
General complaints	Weight gain; fatigue
Urine output	Oliguria
Cardiovascular	Edema, soft and pitting (periorbital, external genitalia, peritoneal and pleural spaces, extremities)
Gastrointestinal	Anorexia; nausea; vomiting

2 DIAGNOSE

NURSING DIAGNOSIS	SUBJECTIVE FINDINGS	OBJECTIVE FINDINGS
Altered renal tissue perfusion related to altered glomerular cells causing proteinuria	None	Foamy urine; protein found in urine by dipstick; decrease in serum protein, albumin, and calcium
Fluid volume excess related to decreased vascular oncotic pressure caused by proteinuria and inadequate protein replacement by the liver	Complains of dyspnea	Increased weight; intake greater than output; blood pressure and pulse normal or slightly increased; edema obvious with jugular venous distention (if edema is severe, central venous pressure and pulmonary artery wedge pressure may be high)
Altered nutrition: less than body requirements related to proteinuria, anorexia, nausea, and vomiting	Complains of fatigue; may complain of anorexia, nausea, vomiting, and metallic taste in mouth	Proteinuria evidenced by dipstick readings; patient states that food tastes bad and refuses to eat
Potential for bathing/hygiene, toileting self-care deficit related to bed rest during acute phase of illness	Complains of fatigue	Bed rest is ordered by physician
Potential for infection related to altered immune process due to lowered serum protein levels or immunosuppressive drugs	None	Signs and symptoms of infection in urinary tract, lungs, or elsewhere

→ ❯ ❯

NURSING DIAGNOSIS	SUBJECTIVE FINDINGS	OBJECTIVE FINDINGS
Potential for impaired skin integrity related to edema	May complain of discomfort in edematous areas	Excoriation, maceration, and infection may be observed
Potential for body image disturbance related to excessive edema and the side effects of drugs	Complains about and shows preoccupation with appearance	Obvious change in appearance caused by edema or side effects of drugs such as corticosteroids

3 PLAN

Patient goals

1. The patient will demonstrate normal serum and urine components.
2. The patient will demonstrate normal fluid balance.
3. The patient will demonstrate adequate nutritional intake.
4. The patient will be able to resume self-care.
5. The patient will be free of infection.
6. The patient will have no impairment of skin integrity.
7. The patient will return to usual appearance or demonstrate adjustment to changes.
8. The patient will be knowledgeable about nephrotic syndrome, its cause and treatment, possible relapse, follow-up care, and the possibility of dialysis or transplantation in the future.

4 IMPLEMENT

NURSING DIAGNOSIS	NURSING INTERVENTIONS	RATIONALE
Altered renal tissue perfusion related to altered glomerular cells causing proteinuria	Assess blood pressure, pulse, and respirations q 6-8 h; assess abdomen, back, and extremities for ascites, anasarca, or peripheral edema.	To identify hypervolemia.
	Monitor urine: protein, specific gravity	Proteinuria may vary with circadian rhythm (high: 4 PM; low: 3 AM).
	Monitor serum protein, albumin, and calcium; Hct	To help determine replacement needed; decreased serum protein means decreased protein-bound calcium.
	Monitor sodium, potassium, chloride, and serum pH	Levels may be lowered with vigorous diuretic therapy
	Monitor BUN and serum creatinine.	To monitor renal function.
	Administer immunosuppressive agents as ordered; monitor response to drugs.	To decrease protein excretion; monitor to determine effectiveness of agent, dosage, and timing, and observe for adverse side effects.

NURSING DIAGNOSIS	NURSING INTERVENTIONS	RATIONALE
Fluid volume excess related to decreased vascular oncotic pressure caused by proteinuria and inadequate protein replacement by the liver	Assess weight daily; also 24-h intake and output; assess blood pressure, pulse, and respirations (sitting and standing) q 6-8 h; monitor edema, jugular venous distention and, as necessary, central venous pressure and pulmonary artery wedge pressure; monitor laboratory data: urine specific gravity, protein; serum albumin, calcium; Hct	To check for altered fluid status, orthostatic hypotension.
	Monitor serum sodium, potassium, chloride, and pH.	Levels may be lowered by vigorous diuretic therapy.
	Administer drugs as ordered (i.e., diuretics, albumin); monitor response to drugs.	To correct fluid imbalance; to determine effect of drugs and to observe for side effects such as hypokalemia and ototoxicity.
	Limit sodium intake as ordered.	If serum levels are high, edema will be worsened by fluid retention.
	Restrict fluid intake as ordered.	May be necessary in cases of hyponatremia, massive edema or ascites, respiratory distress, or pleural effusion.
Altered nutrition: less than body requirements related to proteinuria, anorexia, nausea, and vomiting	Assess food intake.	To ensure adequate intake within the limits prescribed.
	Monitor dry weight.	To determine if weight changes are related to fluid balance or inadequate caloric intake and loss of muscle mass.
	Monitor laboratory data: serum protein, lipids, potassium, and calcium.	To determine whether protein intake is adequate.
	Encourage food intake as prescribed.	Prescribed diet may include increased protein to increase protein synthesis and avoid a negative nitrogen balance; an adequate intake of carbohydrates to prevent use of body proteins for energy; optimum levels of potassium, calcium, and calories as needed; no cholesterol or saturated fats as long as serum lipids are elevated.
	Provide palatable meals, considering patient's likes and dislikes; encourage small, frequent meals; provide oral hygiene before meals; offer hard candy.	To increase intake of needed foods.
	Administer protein supplements if ordered.	Protein intake needed may be hard to achieve by foods alone.
	Refer complex or problem situations to dietitian.	A team approach to managing the complex renal diet is helpful to all concerned.

NURSING DIAGNOSIS	NURSING INTERVENTIONS	RATIONALE
Potential for bathing/hygiene, toileting, self-care deficit related to bed rest during acute phase of illness	Assess need for assistance; assist with self-care as needed; encourage deep breathing, coughing and turning; increase activity as tolerated.	To prevent unwanted side effects of bed rest.
Potential for infection related to altered immune process due to lowered serum protein level or immunosuppressive drugs	Assess for signs and symptoms of infection in secretions, excretions. Monitor laboratory data: WBC.	To detect any infection early. May be lowered in patients taking immunosuppressive drugs, may not be increased with infection.
	Monitor temperature q 4-6 h.	Corticosteroids may mask usual temperature increase with infection.
	Wash hands thoroughly and consistently; avoid exposing patient to individuals with infection.	To decrease chances for infection.
	Ensure aseptic technique for any invasive procedure or wound care.	To decrease chances of infection.
	Encourage regular oral hygiene, hand washing, and bathing, and adequate rest and nutrition.	Good health habits help to prevent infections.
Potential for impaired skin integrity related to edema	Assess skin in edematous areas; provide meticulous care to these areas (skin folds, joint creases, genital areas, back).	Such areas are easily injured, especially skin-to-skin areas.
	Elevate edematous genitalia and extremities.	To prevent excoriation, maceration, or infection.
Potential for body image disturbance related to excessive edema and the side effects of drugs	Warn patient to expect alopecia or other drug side effects and changes caused by edema.	Temporary side effects of drugs and recurrence of edema may change appearance.
	Assess for evidence that change in appearance is a problem.	Early intervention may prevent patient distress.
Knowledge deficit	See Patient Teaching.	

5 EVALUATE

PATIENT OUTCOME	DATA INDICATING THAT OUTCOME IS REACHED
Glomerular function is normal.	Patient has normal serum albumin and lipid levels and urine components.
Fluid balance is normal.	Urine volume is normal and balances intake.
Nutritional status is normal.	Patient has no restrictions on food or fluids.
Patient has resumed self-care.	Patient has no restrictions on ADL.
No infection is present.	Patient has no signs or symptoms of infection.
Skin is intact.	Patient has no areas of excoriation or maceration.
Patient has no problem with body image.	Patient has returned to previous appearance or has adjusted to alteration.
Patient is knowledgeable about nephrotic syndrome.	Patient can explain causes of nephrotic syndrome, possible relapse, need for long-term medical supervision, and possible need for dialysis or transplantation in the future.

PATIENT TEACHING

1. Explain the causes of nephrotic syndrome and its signs, symptoms, and pathophysiology.
2. Explain any diet prescription and medications ordered, and teach self-care skills such as monitoring blood pressure and collecting urine specimens.
3. Describe complications of nephrotic syndrome and how to prevent them.
4. Explain the possibility of relapse and the follow-up medical care needed for monitoring possible changes in renal function.
5. Explain the possible need for dialysis and transplantation in the future.

CHAPTER 9

Cancer and the Kidney

Renal Cell Carcinoma

Renal cell carcinoma is a malignant tumor of the kidneys arising from tubular epithelium.

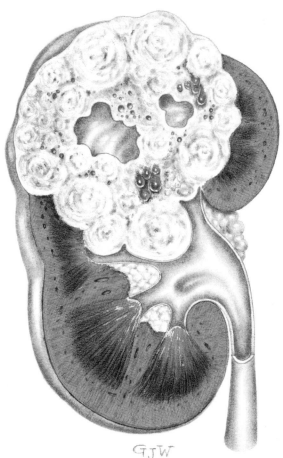

Renal cell carcinoma accounts for 90% of kidney cancers.[8] It is estimated that in 1989, 23,000 cases were diagnosed, and 10,000 people died of the disorder. Renal cell carcinoma occurs most frequently in adult men, with the peak occurrence in the sixth decade of life. The life expectancy of a patient with metastases at the time of diagnosis is poor; only 5% to 20% are alive at the end of 1 year.[6] The disorder usually is unilateral, with equal incidence in the right and left kidneys. There is little evidence for specific carcinogens, although tobacco use appears to be associated with development of the tumor.

PATHOPHYSIOLOGY

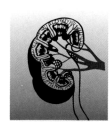

The tumor may arise anywhere in the kidney, and its increasing mass may compress surrounding tissue, causing ischemia, necrosis, and hemorrhage. The tumor may invade the collecting system and branches of the renal vein, even extending into the inferior vena cava. Although the tumor grows slowly, metastases can occur at any stage. Primary sites of metastases are the lungs, lymph nodes, liver, and bones. Renal cell carcinoma

For a photograph of renal cell carcinoma, see Color Plate 8 on page xi.

metastasizes to all visceral organs. Such involvement may be discovered first, and metastases may occur long after the original tumor has been removed.

COMPLICATIONS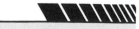

Metastases to the lungs, lymph nodes, liver, and bones

DIAGNOSTIC STUDIES AND FINDINGS

Diagnostic Test	Findings
Laboratory tests	
Complete blood cell count	Normochromic, normocytic anemia or polycythemia caused by an increase in erythropoietin
Erythrocyte sedimentation rate	Elevated
Urinalysis	Hematuria
Kidney-ureter-bladder (KUB) x-ray	Space-occupying lesion
Intravenous urogram	Hypervascular areas
Ultrasonography	Distinguishes between solid mass and cyst
Arteriogram	Details renal vascular anatomy before surgery to detect spread up renal vein
Computed tomography (CT) or magnetic resonance imaging (MRI) scan	Scans of chest, liver, and bone rule out metastases and help stage for tumor
Renal biopsy	Tissue for cytology

MEDICAL MANAGEMENT

GENERAL MANAGEMENT

Efforts are made to stage the tumor's development. No radiation or chemotherapy has been found to effect a cure.

SURGERY

A radical extrafascial nephrectomy may be done, which involves removing the kidney and tumor, neural and vascular structures at the kidney's hilum, surrounding perinephric fat, Gerota's fascia, and the ipsilateral adrenal gland. The prognosis is poor if there is involvement of the renal vein or extension through Gerota's fascia, extension to the renal lymph nodes or contiguous organs, or distant metastases. The need for nephrectomy depends on the severity of symptoms. Radical nephrectomy is not indicated if there is preoperative evidence of local node involvement or advanced disease. A partial nephrectomy is done if the patient has only one kidney. Staging involves examining local nodes and identifying distant metastases.

1 ASSESS

ASSESSMENT	OBSERVATIONS
Abdomen	Mass felt in flank; renal bruit
General complaints	Chronic aching pain in flank; unexplained weight loss

2 DIAGNOSE

NURSING DIAGNOSIS	SUBJECTIVE FINDINGS	OBJECTIVE FINDINGS
Pain related to compression of tissues surrounding tumor	Complains of aching in flank	Guarding behavior
Anticipatory grieving related to perceived potential loss of kidney associated with cancer and its threat to life	Expresses sorrow, feelings of loss	Weeping; altered sleep patterns

3 PLAN

Patient goals

1. The patient will be free of pain.
2. The patient will participate in constructive anticipatory grief work.

3. The patient will be knowledgeable about renal cell carcinoma, its treatment, and follow-up medical care.

4 IMPLEMENT

NURSING DIAGNOSIS	NURSING INTERVENTIONS	RATIONALE
Pain related to compression of tissues surrounding tumor	Assess for pain; give medications for pain as ordered.	To determine need for analgesia; to assess effectiveness of drug, timing, and dosage and to observe for adverse reactions.
Anticipatory grieving related to perceived potential loss of kidney associated with cancer and its threat to life	Encourage patient to express fears and concerns.	To help patient sort out the meaning of the loss.
	Assess previous problem-solving abilities; evaluate support available from family and significant others.	To determine their impact on this event.
	Evaluate need for referral to other services.	Needs may be beyond the nurse's role.
Knowledge deficit	See Patient Teaching.	

5   EVALUATE

PATIENT OUTCOME	DATA INDICATING OUTCOME IS REACHED
Patient is free of pain.	No pain is reported.
Patient is realistic in anticipating the future.	Patient talks about diagnosis and treatment options and uses appropriate resources; constructive interpersonal relationships continue.

PATIENT TEACHING

1. Explain renal cell carcinoma, its treatment, and follow-up medical care.
2. Explain pain-relieving measures.
3. Discuss the need for a balanced, nutritious diet.
4. Discuss changes that should be reported to the physician.

Metastatic Renal Disease

Metastatic renal disease involves a tumor that develops at a site distant from the primary site because of seeding through a body cavity or through lymphatic or hematogenous spread.

Metastases from solid tumors, most frequently in a lung or breast, are isolated events that have little effect on renal function (they may cause painless, intermittent hematuria). Lymphomas and leukemias, however, infiltrate the kidneys, causing swelling, tenderness, and acute renal failure.

THE EFFECTS OF CANCER TREATMENT

The kidneys are subject to the adverse side effects of the treatments used for cancer. Many chemotherapeutic agents are nephrotoxic and cause acute tubular necrosis, acute interstitial nephritis, intratubular urate deposits, or hemolytic-uremic syndrome. (See "Acute Renal Failure," page 37.) It is important to avoid the cumulative effect of a series of treatments with nephrotoxic agents. Protective measures such as adequate hydration and diuresis before giving the drug are examples of such measures.

The kidneys are relatively sensitive to radiation. Extreme care must be taken to limit their exposure. If doses to one kidney above its tolerance are required, efforts are made to spare the other kidney. The effects of radiation to the back or abdomen may cause renal injury that appears after a latent period. Acute renal damage may be manifested as hemolytic-uremic syndrome. Chronic renal failure from progressive fibrosis may be found years later.

RENAL TOXICITY AND CANCER DRUGS

Directly nephrotoxic drugs causing acute tubular necrosis

Cisplatin (Platinol)
Carmustine (also BCNU): BiCNU
Lomustine (CeeNU)
Methotrexate (Amethopterin)
Doxorubicin (Adriamycin)

Directly nephrotoxic drugs causing acute interstitial nephritis

Mercaptopurine (6MP)

Indirect toxicity

Tumor lysis syndrome
Hemolysis and acute renal failure
    Mitomycin (also Mitomycin-C): Mutamycin
    Fluorouracil (5 Fluorouracil)

CHAPTER 10

Obstructive and Congenital Disorders

Hydronephrosis

Hydronephrosis is the dilation of the renal pelvis by the pressure of urine that cannot flow past an obstruction in the urinary tract.

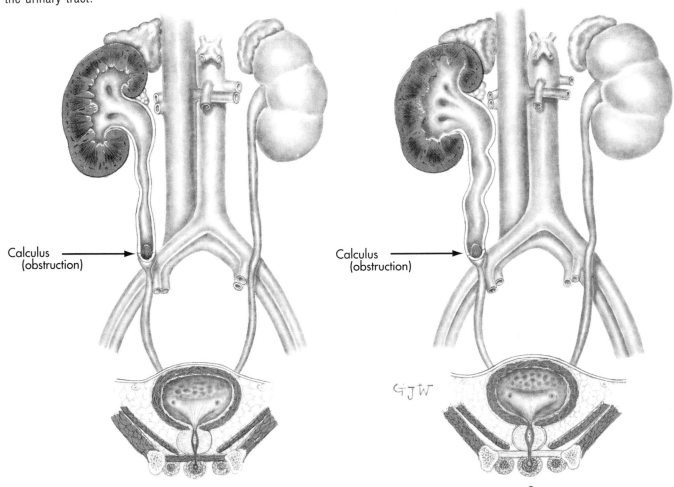

Calculus (obstruction)

Calculus (obstruction)

GJW

1

2

PROGRESSIVE CHANGES IN UNILATERAL HYDRONEPHROSIS

Obstruction can be proximal to the bladder or can occur below the level of the bladder. Hydronephrosis, which usually occurs on the right side, always occurs during pregnancy because of the obstruction caused by the enlarged uterus.

PATHOPHYSIOLOGY

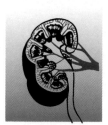

Obstruction of the ureter that results in hydronephrosis may be caused by renal calculi, tumors, inflammation associated with infection, fibrous bands that obstruct the ureteropelvic junction, or prostatic valves. The renal pelvis and ureter dilate and hypertrophy. The pressure of the urine, if prolonged, causes fibrosis and loss of function in the nephrons affected. The duration and severity of the obstruction are significant. Compression causes ischemia and then atrophy of renal tissue. The kidney may be destroyed without pain.

DIAGNOSTIC STUDIES AND FINDINGS

Diagnostic Test	Findings
Renal ultrasonography	Dilation of collecting system
Intravenous urogram	Calyceal clubbing; elongation and dilation of ureter; if obstruction is unilateral, contralateral kidney is larger

COMPLICATIONS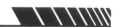

Urinary tract infection
Renal failure

For a photograph of hydronephrosis, see Color Plate 9 on page xi.

MEDICAL MANAGEMENT

GENERAL MANAGEMENT

Management usually is conservative if the condition is not severe.

DRUG THERAPY

Antiinfective agents are used to treat any infection present.

SURGERY

Surgery is performed to relieve the obstruction and preserve renal function. Pyeloplasty or repair of the ureteropelvic junction may be indicated. A nephrectomy may be necessary if the kidney is severely damaged. (See "Kidney Surgery," page 165.)

1 ASSESS

ASSESSMENT	OBSERVATIONS
General complaints	Dull backache; fever with infection
Urinary tract	Hematuria; pyuria
Abdomen	Kidney may be palpable

2 DIAGNOSE

NURSING DIAGNOSIS	SUBJECTIVE FINDINGS	OBJECTIVE FINDINGS
Potential altered renal tissue perfusion related to increased pressure within urine channel because of obstruction at some point in the urinary tract	None	Abdominal mass may be felt
Potential for infection related to urinary tract obstruction	Complains of urgency, dysuria, and frequency	Fever; chills; pyuria; hematuria
Impaired skin integrity related to surgery	None	Incision
Pain related to surgical incision	Complains of discomfort at site of incision; dull ache in loin or costovertebral angle	Guarding behavior

3 PLAN

Patient goals

1. The patient will demonstrate normal renal function without obstruction.
2. The patient will have no infection.
3. The patient will have a healed incision.
4. The patient will be free of pain.
5. The patient will be knowledgeable about hydronephrosis and the need for continuing follow-up care.

→ ❯ ❯

4 IMPLEMENT

NURSING DIAGNOSIS	NURSING INTERVENTIONS	RATIONALE
Potential altered renal tissue perfusion related to increased pressure within urine channel because of obstruction	Assess blood pressure q 6-8 h, 24-h intake and output; weigh daily. Monitor laboratory data: serum creatinine, BUN, serum sodium, potassium, bicarbonate.	Postobstructive diuresis may occur; acute renal failure may develop.
Potential for infection related to urinary tract obstruction	Assess for signs and symptoms of urinary tract infection (fever, increased WBC, pyuria, bacteriuria, foul-smelling urine).	Likelihood of infection is increased with obstruction.
	Administer antiinfective agents as ordered; monitor response to drugs given.	To treat any infection present and to determine response to drug.
Impaired skin integrity related to surgery	Prepare for surgery. (See "Kidney Surgery," page 165). After surgery, assess site of incision for drainage and signs of infection.	To detect any complications promptly.
	Keep area clean and dry.	To avoid skin breakdown and promote healing.
	Keep any drainage tubes patent, unkinked, and anchored; care for urethral catheter.	To maintain urine flow and to avoid inadvertent displacement. Tubes may include a stent (a catheter inserted into the ureter), a nephrostomy tube, and a drain in the incision; drainage from the incision may continue for several days.
Pain related to surgical incision	Assess for discomfort and give analgesics as ordered. Monitor and record response to drug.	To determine the need for pain relief and to relieve discomfort. To determine effectiveness of drug, dosage, and timing and any side effects.
	Report any pain that occurs after the immediate postoperative period.	Pain with fever and decreased urine output may indicate obstruction or leakage of urine into the retroperitoneal space.
Knowledge deficit	See Patient Teaching.	

5 EVALUATE

PATIENT OUTCOME	DATA INDICATING THAT OUTCOME IS REACHED
Obstruction is relieved; renal function is normal.	X-rays show hydronephrosis is lessened or has not increased; renal function tests are normal or stable.
No infection is present in the urinary tract.	Patient has no signs or symptoms of urinary tract infection.
Incision is healing.	No drainage, redness, swelling, or separation of incision is noted.
Patient is pain free.	Patient does not complain of pain.
Patient and family are knowledgeable about hydronephrosis.	Patient and family understand the condition and the need for follow-up medical care.

PATIENT TEACHING ■

1. Explain the kidney-ureter abnormality.
2. Explain possible problems, i.e., recurrent infection and obstruction.
3. Explain signs and symptoms of urinary tract infection and obstruction.
4. Explain measures to prevent urinary tract infections, such as adequate fluid intake to avoid dehydration, regular emptying of bladder to avoid overdistention, and good perineal hygiene to prevent microorganisms from entering the urinary tract.
5. Explain postoperative care, including care of the incision and self-monitoring skills as needed.
6. Explain plans for follow-up medical care and monitoring of renal function.

Polycystic kidney disease

Polycystic kidney disease is a disorder in which the kidney tissue is replaced by grapelike clusters of cysts.

For a photograph of polycystic kidney disease, see Color Plate 10, page xi.

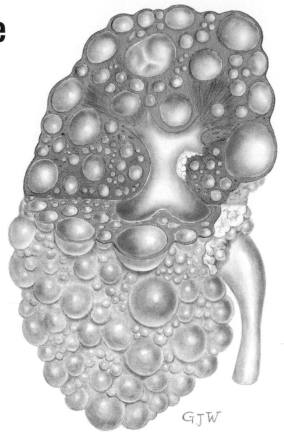

Polycystic kidney disease (PKD) is a genetically transmitted disorder (autosomal dominant in adults). An infant form (autosomal recessive) occurs, but these children rarely live more than a year. The adult form of the disease has a similar onset, clinical course, and manifestations within a family. Approximately 5% to 10% of all patients on dialysis have the adult form of PKD. It is important that the cysts characteristic of PKD be differentiated from tumors. Fifteen percent of patients with polycystic kidney disease may have an associated berry aneurysm with the possibility of subarachnoid hemorrhage. The incidence of polycystic kidney disease is 1 in 1,000.[24]

PATHOPHYSIOLOGY

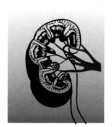

In polycystic kidney disease, normal kidney tissue is replaced by grapelike clusters of cysts that enlarge over time and destroy the surrounding tissue by compression. Why the cysts form is not clear. They may be associated with cysts in the liver. The cysts may occur anywhere along the nephron, and they are filled with a yellow or brown fluid that may be thick and cloudy and may contain urine components. Progressive fibrosis of the interstitial tissue occurs. Infection and renal stones often develop because of urinary stasis and compression. Ascending infection may become a persistent source of infection. These kidneys do not resist infection well and thus may harbor organisms; poor perfusion may prevent antibiotics from reaching pockets of infection. A perinephric abscess may form, and septicemia may occur. In these cases a nephrectomy may be necessary. Hypertension and renal failure follow the onset of symptoms within 5 to 15 years.

COMPLICATIONS

Berry aneurysm	Renal bleeding
Subarachnoid hemorrhage	Obstruction
Infection	Malignancy
Calculi	Salt-wasting defect
Liver cysts	

CONGENITAL ANOMALIES

A wide variety of anomalies related to the kidneys can occur. The abnormalities may be in number, volume, form, location, or rotation and may involve the blood vessels, renal pelvis, or ureter. Errors in renal development result from failure to develop, abnormal division of the elements, fusion of the elements, or abnormal movement from the pelvic to the lumbar area. These anatomic deviations may range from minor to severe and from easily correctable to incompatible with life. Renal abnormalities are frequently associated with other irregular conditions such as low-set ears, imperforate anus, genital abnormalities, and abnormalities of the spinal cord and extremities.

DIAGNOSTIC STUDIES AND FINDINGS

Diagnostic Test	Findings
Laboratory tests	
Urinalysis	Intermittent hematuria; proteinuria; bacteriuria; pyuria
Renal function tests (serum creatinine, blood urea nitrogen, creatinine clearance)	Function may be decreased
Kidney-ureter-bladder (KUB) x-ray and renal ultrasonography	Enlarged kidneys
Intravenous urogram	Irregular outline and distortion of calyceal pattern; presence of cysts, nephrocalcinosis, or obstruction of the collecting system

MEDICAL MANAGEMENT

GENERAL MANAGEMENT

No specific treatment is available for PKD. Medical goals concentrate on preventing hypertension and infection to preserve renal function. Instrumentation of the urinary tract, which is occasionally followed by a urinary tract infection, should be avoided. If patients do not have symptoms, creatinine clearance and urine cultures should be obtained twice a year. Genetic counseling may be suggested for families with polycystic kidney disease. Renal dialysis and transplantation may be indicated when chronic renal failure ensues.

1 ASSESS

ASSESSMENT	OBSERVATIONS
Abdomen	Palpable kidneys

2 DIAGNOSE

NURSING DIAGNOSIS	SUBJECTIVE FINDINGS	OBJECTIVE FINDINGS
Altered renal tissue perfusion related to replacement of normal renal tissue with cysts	None	Blood pressure may be elevated

NURSING DIAGNOSIS	SUBJECTIVE FINDINGS	OBJECTIVE FINDINGS
Potential for infection related to alterations of the collecting system by cysts	Reports urgency and dysuria	Frequent urination
Pain related to enlarged or infected cysts	Describes pain (dull or sharp) in loins or lateral abdomen	Costovertebral angle or loin tenderness
Potential altered family processes related to diagnosis of a genetically transmitted disease	Patient expresses feelings about possibility of other family members having same problem	

3 PLAN

Patient goals

1. The patient will have stable renal function.
2. The patient will be knowledgeable about measures to prevent urinary tract infections.
3. The patient will be free of pain.
4. The patient and family will be knowledgeable about polycystic kidney disease, its anticipated course, and the necessary medical supervision.

4 IMPLEMENT

NURSING DIAGNOSIS	NURSING INTERVENTIONS	RATIONALE
Altered renal tissue perfusion related to replacement of normal renal tissue with cysts	Assess and monitor intake, output, and weight if necessary.	Renal insufficiency or failure may develop.
	Monitor blood pressure; administer antihypertensive drugs if ordered.	Antihypertensives decrease effect of elevated blood pressure on already damaged kidneys.
	Monitor laboratory data that reflect renal function.	To follow any decrease in renal function.
Potential for infection related to alterations of the collecting system by cysts	Assess for signs and symptoms of urinary tract infection.	Cysts are prone to infection because of changes they cause in renal blood flow or urine flow.
	Avoid inserting catheters or other instruments into the urinary tract.	To prevent nosocomial infection.

NURSING DIAGNOSIS	NURSING INTERVENTIONS	RATIONALE
Pain related to enlarged or infected cysts	Assess patient's need for pain relief.	Enlarged, infected cysts may cause discomfort.
	Administer analgesic drug as ordered and monitor response to drug; apply external heat to lumbar area.	To help relieve discomfort.
Potential altered family processes related to diagnosis of a genetically transmitted disease	Assess how diagnosis of patient's condition affects others in family.	To determine need for family counseling.
	Provide information about genetic counseling if appropriate.	Some people do not want to know this information.
Knowledge deficit	See Patient Teaching.	

5 EVALUATE

PATIENT OUTCOME	DATA INDICATING THAT OUTCOME IS REACHED
Early decreases in renal function are recognized.	Urinalysis and blood chemistries are performed q 6 mo, and any change is noted.
Infections are treated promptly.	Patient seeks medical help when signs and symptoms of urinary tract infection occur.
Patient is free from pain.	Patient has no complaint of pain.
Patient is knowledgeable and plans are made for long-term treatment.	Patient describes the anticipated course of the disease and the possible relationship of dialysis and transplantation for the future.

PATIENT TEACHING

1. Explain the nature of the kidney abnormality and the availability of genetic counseling (see page 184).
2. Explain the need to monitor renal function and blood pressure.
3. Explain measures to prevent urinary tract infection: adequate fluid intake to avoid dehydration, regular emptying of the bladder to avoid overdistention, observation of urine, and good perineal care to prevent entrance of microorganisms into the urinary tract.
4. Explain signs and symptoms of urinary tract infections (see "Pyelonephritis," page 63).
5. Explain renal dialysis and transplantation as options for the future.

Kidney Displacement and Supernumerary Kidneys

Kidney displacement occurs occasionally when the kidneys do not ascend to their normal positions or when one crosses over, placing both kidneys on one side. A **supernumerary (extra) kidney** rarely occurs, although duplication of the renal pelvis is common.

PATHOPHYSIOLOGY

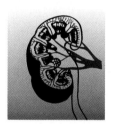

The displaced kidneys may be normal except for their location or rotation. They are more susceptible to trauma, because they are not as well protected as a kidney in its normal location. Obstruction may occur, as may infarction or infection, if the normal blood supply and urinary channel are interrupted. The extra kidney may be small, dysplastic, and infected.

COMPLICATIONS

Traumatic injury
Infection
Infarction

DIAGNOSTIC STUDIES AND FINDINGS

Diagnostic Test	Findings
Intravenous urogram	Abnormally located or rotated kidney; extra kidney

MEDICAL MANAGEMENT

SURGERY

Correction of obstruction to blood supply or urine elimination in displaced kidney and removal of extra kidney may be indicated; the remaining kidney must function adequately. (See "Kidney Surgery," page 165.)

1   ASSESS

ASSESSMENT	OBSERVATIONS
Urinary tract	Asymptomatic or showing signs of infection or obstruction
Renal function	Serum creatinine and BUN may be elevated

2   DIAGNOSE

NURSING DIAGNOSIS	SUBJECTIVE FINDINGS	OBJECTIVE FINDINGS
Potential for infection related to abnormality of blood supply or urine channel	None	Asymptomatic unless infection is present
Impaired skin integrity related to surgery	None	Incision and drainage tubes
Pain related to surgery	Describes pain at site of incision	Guarding behavior

3   PLAN

Patient goals

1. The patient will be free of signs and symptoms of urinary tract infection or obstruction.
2. The patient will have a healed incision after surgery.
3. The patient will be free of pain.
4. The patient will understand possible problems associated with kidney displacement or an extra kidney.

4   IMPLEMENT

NURSING DIAGNOSIS	NURSING INTERVENTIONS	RATIONALE
Potential for infection related to abnormality of blood supply or urine channel	Assess for signs and symptoms of urinary tract infection; monitor temperature, nature of urine.	Abnormal urine channel or blood supply may increase susceptibility to urinary tract infection.
Impaired skin integrity related to surgery	Prepare patient for surgery. (See "Kidney Surgery," page 165.)	
	After surgery, assess site of incision for drainage and signs of infection.	To detect complications promptly.

→ › ›

NURSING DIAGNOSIS	NURSING INTERVENTIONS	RATIONALE
	Keep area clean and dry.	To avoid skin breakdown and promote healing.
	Keep any drainage tubes patent, unkinked, and anchored.	To permit continuous drainage and avoid inadvertent displacement.
	Be alert to and report any foul-smelling urine, pus, or blood.	To detect complications promptly.
Pain related to surgery	Assess patient's need for pain relief; administer analgesic drug as ordered; monitor response.	To determine need for drug, promote patient's comfort, and determine effectiveness of dosage and timing; also to identify any side effects.
Knowledge deficit	See Patient Teaching	

5 EVALUATE

PATIENT OUTCOME	DATA INDICATING THAT OUTCOME IS REACHED
No urinary tract infection is present.	Patient's temperature and WBC are normal; urinalysis has no bacteria or pus cells.
Incision has healed.	Wound is closed, and no infection is present.
Patient is pain free.	Patient does not complain of discomfort.
Patient and family are knowledgeable about patient's condition.	Patient and family can explain the signs of possible problems related to the location of the kidney, measures to prevent urinary tract infections, and any postoperative care needed.

PATIENT TEACHING

1. Explain the location of the displaced or extra kidney(s).
2. Explain the signs and symptoms of possible problems (trauma to the abdomen, urinary tract infections, or urinary tract obstruction).
3. Explain measures to prevent urinary tract infection, such as adequate fluid intake to avoid dehydration, regular emptying of the bladder to avoid overdistention, and good perineal hygiene to prevent microorganisms from entering the urinary tract.
4. Explain postoperative care, including care of the incision and any self-monitoring skill needed.

Hypoplasia and Dysplasia of the Kidney

Hypoplasia is a condition in which fewer than the usual number of nephrons are present. **Dysplasia** is a condition in which areas of the kidney have underdeveloped structures. When these defects occur together, the term used is **hypodysplasia.**

PATHOPHYSIOLOGY

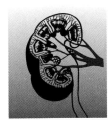

With hypoplasia, the kidneys are small but normal in structure. They may be dysplastic, with malformation of renal tissue. If both kidneys are severely malformed, death occurs in the neonatal period. One kidney usually has poorer function than the other.

COMPLICATIONS

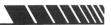

Urinary tract infection
Renal failure

DIAGNOSTIC STUDIES AND FINDINGS

Diagnostic Test	Findings
Intravenous urogram	Small, malformed kidney(s)

MEDICAL MANAGEMENT

GENERAL MANAGEMENT

Chronic renal failure may ensue. (See "Renal Dialysis," page 135.)

DRUG THERAPY

Antiinfective agents may be needed for urinary tract infection.

SURGERY

Elective surgical removal of the dysplastic kidney usually is performed. Careful assessment of the contralateral kidney is essential. If chronic renal failure occurs, transplantation may be undertaken, if technically feasible. (See "Renal Transplantation," page 157.)

1 ASSESS

ASSESSMENT	OBSERVATIONS
Renal function	May be asymptomatic; bilateral involvement: uremia; unilateral involvement: infection, hypertension, or renal failure

2 DIAGNOSE

NURSING DIAGNOSIS	SUBJECTIVE FINDINGS	OBJECTIVE FINDINGS
Impaired skin integrity related to surgery	None	Incision and drainage tubes
Pain related to surgery	Describes pain at site of incision	Guarding behavior
Potential for infection related to abnormality of urine channel	None	Asymptomatic unless infection is present

3 PLAN

Patient goals

1. The patient will demonstrate prompt recovery from any surgery performed.
2. The patient will be free of pain.
3. The patient will be free of any signs or symptoms of urinary tract infection.
4. The patient will describe possible problems associated with kidney hypoplasia or dysplasia.

4 IMPLEMENT

NURSING DIAGNOSIS	NURSING INTERVENTIONS	RATIONALE
Impaired skin integrity related to surgery	Prepare patient for surgery. (See "Kidney Surgery," page 165.)	
	After surgery, monitor site of incision for drainage and signs of infection.	To detect any complications promptly.
	Keep area clean and dry.	To avoid skin breakdown and promote healing.
	Keep any drainage tubes patent, unkinked, and anchored; care for urethral catheter.	To permit continuous drainage and avoid inadvertent displacement; tubes may include a drain in the incision.

NURSING DIAGNOSIS	NURSING INTERVENTIONS	RATIONALE
	Report any foul-smelling urine, blood, or pus in drainage.	Such complications may follow surgery.
Pain related to surgery	Assess patient's need for pain relief; administer analgesic as ordered; monitor response.	To determine need for analgesic, to promote comfort, to determine drug's effectiveness in timing and dosage, and to identify any side effects.
	Assist with personal hygiene as needed after surgery.	Pain may interfere with self-care.
Potential for infection related to abnormality of urine channel	Assess for signs and symptoms of urinary tract infection; monitor temperature, WBC, problems with urination, and urine (bacteria, pus cells).	Infection may occur in the urinary tract after surgery.
Knowledge deficit	See Patient Teaching	

5 EVALUATE

PATIENT OUTCOME	DATA INDICATING THAT OUTCOME IS REACHED
Patient has recovered from surgery.	Incision is healed.
Patient is free of pain.	Patient does not complain of discomfort.
Patient has no infection.	No signs or symptoms of urinary tract infection are noted.
Patient and family are knowledgeable about patient's condition.	Patient and family can describe the renal abnormality and its implications.

PATIENT TEACHING

1. Explain the kidney's abnormality.
2. Explain the possible problems, i.e., urinary tract infection, renal failure, and their signs and symptoms.
3. Describe measures to prevent urinary tract infection, such as adequate fluid intake to avoid dehydration, regular emptying of the bladder to avoid overdistention, and good perineal hygiene to prevent microorganisms from entering the urinary tract.
4. Explain postoperative care, including care of incision and any self-monitoring skills needed.
5. Explain that renal dialysis and transplantation are likely future options in the event of chronic renal failure.

CHAPTER 11

Surgical and Therapeutic Procedures

Hemodialysis

Hemodialysis involves circulating the patient's blood through semipermeable tubing that is surrounded by a dialysate solution in the artificial kidney (Figure 11-1). It replaces part of the kidney's normal function.

The blood circuit includes an access device (cannula or internal arteriovenous fistula); arterial blood lines (with blood pressure monitor); a blood pump; a dialyzer, where diffusion, osmosis, and ultrafiltration occur; and venous lines with filter and monitors (for clots or air emboli and pressure), which return blood to the patient.

The dialysis circuit includes a supply of dialysate concentrate and a supply of treated water, which are combined by a proportioning pump so that the desired concentration is delivered to the dialyzer; monitors that detect the pressure, concentration, and temperature of the dialysate and stop the flow of dialysate if preset levels are not met; a dialyzer, where the dialysate accepts wastes, excess electrolytes, and water; dialysate exit lines, which may have a leak detector (blood-in-effluent lines) or are monitored using Hemastix to detect the presence of blood; a negative pressure gauge on the di-alysate lines that controls ultrafiltration; and a bypass circuit for diversion of dialysate that is not within the preset temperature, conductivity, or pressure limits.

The composition of the diluted dialysate solution is sodium, 130 to 145 mEq/L; potassium, 0 to 3 mEq/L; calcium, 2.5 to 4 mEq/L; chloride, 96 to 107 mEq/L; and acetate, 33 to 41 mEq/L. Bicarbonate may be used in place of acetate.

Blood access is achieved by means of an internal arteriovenous fistula created surgically with the patient's artery and vein, endogenous vein grafts, exogenous vein (bovine) grafts, or grafts made of artificial material such as expanded polytetrafluorethylene or by means of an external arteriovenous shunt or cannula (Figure 11-2).

Hemodialysis treatment schedules vary with the kind of machine used and the patient's condition. Treatments are usually scheduled three times a week for 3 to 6 hours each.

The major types of artificial kidneys are hollow fiber and flat plate (Figure 11-3). The hollow fiber kidney is increasingly used because it can be adapted to the size of the patient. In the hollow fiber kidney, the blood flows through narrow filaments that are surrounded by dialysate. In the flat-plate kidney, the blood and dialysate flow in opposite directions in alternate layers.

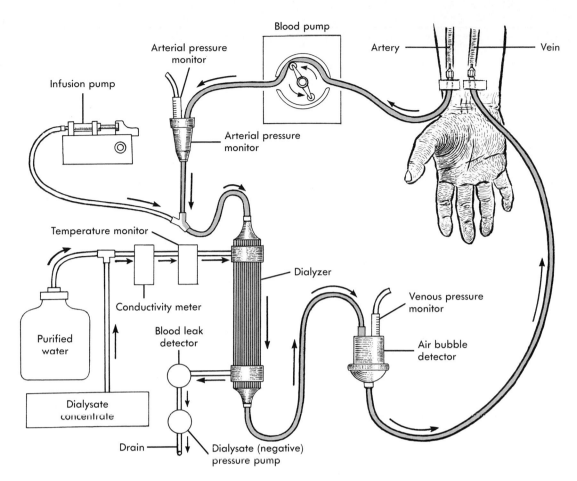

FIGURE 11-1
Components of a hemodialysis system. (From Thelan.[26])

RENAL DIALYSIS

Dialysis is the differential diffusion of permeable substances through a semipermeable membrane separating two solutions. **Hemodialysis** and **peritoneal dialysis** are two forms of dialysis used clinically to treat patients with acute or chronic renal failure. The dialysate fluid contains electrolytes similar to those in normal blood plasma to permit diffusion of electrolytes into or out of the patient's blood. Glucose is added to the dialysate fluid to raise the osmolality and remove water from the blood channel.

Dialysis replaces some, but not all, of the kidney's functions. Fluid volume, electrolyte balance, acid-base balance, and nitrogenous wastes are controlled.

Dialysis options include home or in-center hemodialysis, home or in-center intermittent peritoneal dialysis, continuous cycling peritoneal dialysis (CCPD), and continuous ambulatory peritoneal dialysis (CAPD). Dialysis plays an important role in renal transplant programs by providing a backup for failed transplants and a pool of potential transplant recipients.

According to the 1990 report of the U. S. Renal Data System there were 110,253 patients on dialysis at the end of 1988, the latest year for which they report essentially complete statistics. In-center hemodialysis was the most frequently used procedure (N = 83,410). The number of patients using home hemodialysis continues to decline (N = 2757). The use of continuous ambulatory peritoneal dialysis has increased (N = 11,683).[28]

Hemofiltration is an alternative to dialysis. This treatment uses a convective filtration process on a continuous rather than intermittent schedule. Pressure differences in the hemofilter force water and solutes through the highly permeable membrane in proportion to their concentrations in the blood. The ultrafiltrate formed is discarded, and depending on the patient's condition, most of the water and solutes removed are replaced. This procedure is used increasingly in the United States for acute renal failure; in Europe, it is used with a blood pump for patients with chronic renal failure. It is a simple system that uses a percutaneous access. A longer treatment time is required, thus avoiding peaks and valleys in blood chemistry values. Hemofiltration can be combined with hemodialysis in the process known as **hemodiafiltration.**

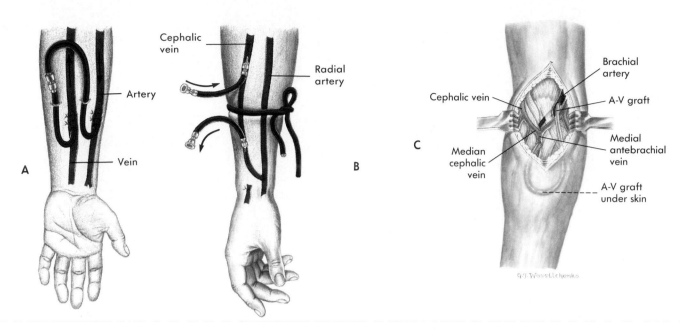

FIGURE 11-2
Circulatory access for hemodialysis. **A,** External (temporary) arteriovenous cannula (shunt). **B,** Internal (permanent) arteriovenous fistula. **C,** Internal (permanent) arteriovenous graft. (**A** and **B** from Thompson[27]; **C** from Thelan.[26])

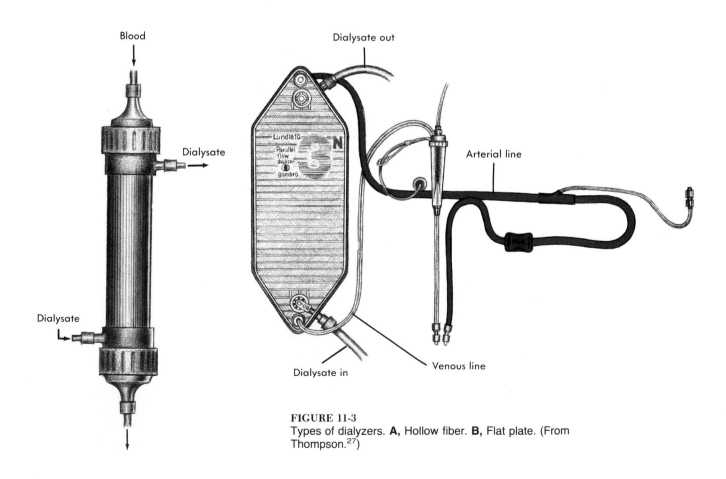

FIGURE 11-3
Types of dialyzers. **A,** Hollow fiber. **B,** Flat plate. (From Thompson.[27])

INDICATIONS

Need for rapid, efficient treatment:
  Acute poisoning (aspirin, methanol, phenobarbital)
  Acute renal failure
  Chronic renal failure
  Severe edema states
  Hepatic coma
  Metabolic acidosis
  Extensive burns with prerenal azotemia
  Transfusion reactions
  Postpartum renal insufficiency
  Crush syndrome

CONTRAINDICATIONS AND CAUTIONS

Other major chronic illness
No vascular access
Hemorrhagic diathesis
Extremes of age
Inability to cooperate with treatment regimen

COMPLICATIONS

  Hemodynamic problems
    Bleeding
    Clot formation
    Hypovolemia
    Hypervolemia
    Angina
    Dysrhythmias
    Anemia
  Infection
    Vascular access site
    Pyrogenic reactions
    Hepatitis B
  Metabolic problems
    Dialysis disequilibrium
    Dialysis dementia
  Mechanical problems
    Membrane rupture
    Failure of temperature, pressure, osmolality, and bubble monitors
    Loosened connections
    Shunt or fistula failure
    Hemolysis
    Air embolism

MEDICAL MANAGEMENT

Anemia, hypertension, infection, peripheral neuropathy, pericarditis, renal osteodystrophy, reproductive dysfunction, and psychosocial difficulties associated with uremia continue to require treatment (see "Chronic Renal Failure," page 49). The goal of therapy is to delay end-stage renal disease by conservative management and to begin dialysis or perform renal transplant at the appropriate point in the course of the disease. Drug dosages and intervals must be modified when the kidney is involved in the drug's excretion. Rates of excretion and metabolism and sensitivity to drugs may be altered.

GENERAL MANAGEMENT

Medical management between dialyses includes: diet: low protein (1 g/kg/day, 50% high biologic value); low sodium (1,500-2,000 mg or 65-85 mEq/day); low potassium (1,560-2,760 mg or 40-70 mEq/day); calories (35 kcal/kg ideal body weight/day); fluids restricted (0.5-1 L/day); a specific amount is determined by the patient's dry weight (weight at which, after dialysis, patient has normal volume relationships).

DRUG THERAPY

Anticoagulants (to prevent normal clotting activated when blood contacts surfaces of blood tubing and dialyzer): Heparin sodium, systemic by injection or continuous infusion; regional by adding drug to the blood line as it enters the dialyzer, then neutralizing it with protamine sulfate as it exits the machine and before it returns to the patient.

Antihypertensive agents: Omit on day of dialysis.

Vitamins (water soluble): To replace those lost during dialysis.

DIALYZER REUSE

To keep costs down, dialyzers are sometimes reused. This requires careful rinsing and resterilization of the equipment. Possible complications include pyrogenic reactions, bacteremia, membrane rupture, and occlusion of hollow fibers.

HEMODIALYSIS MONITORS

Each machine has visible and audible alarms that signal problems outside the preset upper and lower limits and cause portions of the system to be shut off or bypassed.

Dialysate compartment
  Temperature: Measures and controls level
  Flow rate: Reflects fluctuations in rate
  Conductivity: Detects hyperosmolality or hypoosmolality
  Pressure: Detects high or low levels
  Blood leak: Detects blood in dialysate as it leaves the machine (membrane rupture)

Blood compartment
  Pressure: Arterial and venous lines (stops blood pump)
  Air bubbles: Detects air in venous line (stops blood pump and clamps venous line)

WATER TREATMENT

Water used in dialysis must be treated to remove substances toxic to the patient or harmful to the machine. Treatment methods include filtration, softening, deionization, reverse osmosis, and distillation. This removes dissolved anions or cations (sodium, chloride, iron, magnesium, manganese, copper, nitrates, fluoride, and iodide) and organic materials (chloramines, pyrogens, and endotoxins). Bacteria do not cross the dialyzer membrane unless there is a leak. Bacterial growth in dialysate may change the pH, decrease the glucose concentration, and release toxins that cause chills, nausea, vomiting, and fever.

PROCEDURAL GUIDELINES

Before hemodialysis

1. Measure and record for baseline data: temperature, pulse, respirations, and blood pressure (both lying and standing).
2. Review pretreatment blood urea nitrogen; serum creatinine, sodium, and potassium levels; and hematocrit. Be aware of infections with hepatitis B virus (HBV) and human immunodeficiency virus (HIV), if known.
3. Check machine to ensure that: (1) machine is plugged in and working properly, (2) dialysate concentration is as ordered, (3) tubing is sterile and patent and all air has been flushed out, (4) the sterilizing agent used (formaldehyde or chlorine bleach) has been removed, (5) all connections are secure, and (6) all monitors have been set.

During hemodialysis

1. Wear mask and have patient wear mask during initiation and discontinuation of dialysis. Wear protective clothing, goggles, apron, and gloves. Use sterile technique for needle insertions and shunt connections, and anchor connections securely. Precautions against infection must be taken for all concerned.
2. Check equipment for readiness, safety, and gauge settings. Monitor vital signs, intake and output, equipment parameters (blood flow rate, pressures, temperature, osmolality, clots, air emboli, negative pressure for ultrafiltration, and blood leaks), and clotting times. Watch for rapid shifts in volume or electrolytes that may result in hypovolemia, angina, dysrhythmias, nausea, and muscle cramps. Minimize blood loss.

After hemodialysis

1. Measure and record vital signs and weight after discontinuing treatment. Use precautions against infection. Provide routine care to shunt or fistula. Avoid trauma to sites. Do not use arm with shunt or fistula for blood pressure readings or needle sticks. Check circulation. Palpate thrill or auscultate venous blood flow. Record blood urea nitrogen and serum creatinine, sodium, and potassium levels to note effects of treatment.

Care between treatments

1. Encourage patient to follow diet and fluid restrictions as ordered; to take medications as ordered; to call nurse or physician as appropriate for problems. Limit weight gain to 0.5 kg/day between treatments. Regular shunt or fistula care is required.

DIALYSIS DISEQUILIBRIUM SYNDROME

Dialysis disequilibrium syndrome may occur near the end of dialysis or after it. The condition is related to the osmotic gradient produced across the blood-brain barrier by the efficient removal of urea from the blood, but not from the brain tissue. The urea draws in water from the extracellular fluid and causes cerebral edema. Other factors that may be involved are changes in serum pH, rapid ion shifts, and cardiovascular changes. The signs and symptoms of disequilibrium syndrome are headache, nausea, vomiting, agitation, twitching, confusion, and seizures. This syndrome can be prevented by slowing the rate of solute removal by dialyzing at a slower blood flow rate (100 ml/minute) and for a shorter time, using a less efficient dialyzer, or using peritoneal dialysis.

DIALYSIS DEMENTIA

Dialysis dementia, or progressive dialysis encephalopathy, is a syndrome that has emerged as experience with hemodialysis has increased. The clinical picture includes disturbed speech that occurs first during dialysis, myoclonus, dementia, or behavioral changes. It is a progressive condition that ends in death. A number of studies have implicated aluminum accumulation from the water supply or from aluminum hydroxide taken as a phosphate binder.

DIALYSIS-ASSOCIATED HEPATITIS B

Dialysis-associated hepatitis B is a major concern for patients (often active carriers of the hepatitis B virus), staff (at risk because of frequent exposure to patient's blood), and families (at risk because of close contact, especially sexual, and from environmental surfaces). It should be noted that special precautions with blood and other bodily fluids are needed to prevent spreading the hepatitis B virus (HBV). Health care professionals and patients in dialysis units are particularly at risk, because a patient with chronic renal failure receives frequent transfusions and may have a subclinical case of hepatitis B infection owing to impairment of the immune system.

The hepatitis B surface antigen (Hb$_s$Ag) is a useful marker for active HBV infections. Transmission occurs by way of some environmental surfaces (toothbrushes, razors, and needles) and by blood, blood products, and other bodily secretions containing serum. The primary sources are infected serum, saliva, and semen. Other sources of HBV can be bile, sweat, tears, breast milk, vaginal secretions, cerebrospinal fluid, synovial fluid, and cord blood.

Programs to prevent the spread of HBV infections focus on identifying persons who are Hb$_s$Ag positive. All dialysis unit personnel and patients are screened regularly. Such programs also include hygienic measures: safe, reliable procedures for handling laboratory specimens; procedures for hepatitis B precautions for hospitalized patients, including safe care of disposable materials, food handling, and laundry service; segregation of equipment used for patients who are Hb$_s$Ag positive; vigilant hand-washing practices; sterilization measures appropriate to the material involved; no eating, smoking, or other hand-to-mouth activity in the dialysis unit or laboratory; use of protective clothing, such as masks, goggles, gloves, aprons, shoe covers, gowns, and caps; and policy of reporting and recording any unusual exposure to HBV.

Hepatitis B vaccine is used for active immunization for preexposure prevention in high-risk groups, such as dialysis unit personnel. Hepatitis B immune globulin is used for passive immunization after exposure to HBV.

BLOOD ACCESS DEVICES

External arteriovenous shunt
Internal arteriovenous fistula
Grafts
Subclavian vein catheter
Femoral vein catheter

CARE OF ACCESS SITES

- Permit no one to take blood pressure or to perform intravenous punctures in arm with fistula or cannula (to prevent infection or clotting).
- Perform regular shunt care. Wear mask and goggles. Inspect exit sites for infection. Cleanse gently with hydrogen peroxide and applicator sticks using aseptic technique. Clean shunt with alcohol sponges, starting at exit site. Cover with dry sterile dressing and hold in place with paper tape and woven gauze bandage.
- Avoid trauma to shunt. Check circulation (palpate thrill) on venous side and check for clots. Instruct patient to wear loose sleeves, avoid temperature extremes or lifting heavy objects, avoid prolonged immersion of arm in water (arm may be temporarily covered with plastic), and carry clamps to stop bleeding if the shunt separates.
- Provide fistula care. Apply direct pressure to needle sites for 5 minutes or until bleeding stops. Cover with Band-Aid. Pressure dressing may be used.
- Watch for signs of bleeding, infection, ischemia of hand, or aneurysm formation. Watch for clotting and formation of scar tissue from repeated venipunctures.

1 ASSESS

ASSESSMENT	OBSERVATIONS
General	Muscle cramps, pruritus
Cardiovascular	Vascular access problems: bleeding, clotting, infection Hypervolemia, hypertension, tachycardia, increased central venous pressure, jugular venous distention, extra heart sound (S3), lung sounds (crackles), postural edema, weight gain Hypovolemia, hypotension, postural changes, tachycardia, flat neck veins, thirst, dry mucous membranes, weight loss
Neurologic	Dialysis disequilibrium syndrome: headache, nausea, vomiting, agitation, twitching, confusion, seizures Dialysis dementia: disturbed speech, myoclonus, dementia (i.e., confusion, personality and cognitive changes)
Psychosocial	Uncooperative, angry, depressed, in denial
Mechanical problems	Hypertonic or hypotonic dialysate, cold or overheated dialysate, air infusion

2 DIAGNOSIS

NURSING DIAGNOSIS	SUPPORTIVE ASSESSMENT FINDINGS
Fluid volume excess related to fluid accumulation since last treatment	Dyspnea, weight gain, elevated blood pressure
Fluid volume deficit related to too rapid fluid removal during treatment and potential blood loss	Nausea, muscle cramps, lowered blood pressure
Potential for infection related to invasive procedure and blood transfusion requirements	Local signs and symptoms at site of shunt exits or fistula needle punctures; systemic signs and symptoms of sepsis, hepatitis
Altered thought processes related to dialysis disequilibrium syndrome or dialysis dementia	Headache, nausea, vomiting, agitation, twitching, confusion, seizures; disturbed speech patterns, myoclonus, dementia
Body image disturbance related to chronic renal failure (CRF) requiring dependence on a machine	Complains of feeling hopeless, helpless; may deny reality or accept need for dialysis; may have less social activity; life-style changes, withdrawal; may have excess concern with losses, depression, self-neglect, noncompliance with regimen, possibility of suicide
Altered family processes related to need for hemodialysis	Expresses sense of loss, inability to continue usual family roles; spouse or significant other describes stresses of situation (disruption, expense, altered time commitments); family withdrawal

3 PLAN

Patient goals

1. The patient will have gained no more than 0.5 kg per day since the last treatment.
2. The patient will undergo dialysis safely, without machine problems or hypotension.
3. The patient will not develop an infection.
4. The patient will have no alteration in thought processes.
5. The patient and family will understand the changes in body image that are part of chronic renal failure requiring hemodialysis.
6. The patient and family will discuss alterations in the family caused by chronic renal failure requiring hemodialysis and seek help appropriately.
7. The patient and family will understand the purpose of hemodialysis, the process involved, the care required between treatments, and relevant concerns about chronic renal failure. (See "Chronic Renal Failure," page 49)

4 IMPLEMENT

NURSING DIAGNOSIS	NURSING INTERVENTIONS	RATIONALE
Fluid volume excess related to fluid accumulation since last treatment	Assess weight, blood pressure, intake and output, respirations, and pulse.	To determine fluid status as a basis for treatment parameters.
	Monitor laboratory values: blood urea nitrogen (BUN); serum creatinine, sodium, potassium, calcium, magnesium, and phosphate levels; hemoglobin and hematocrit.	Nitrogenous wastes and electrolytes accumulate between treatments; anemia is a continuing problem of chronic renal failure (CRF) and blood losses.
Fluid volume deficit related to too rapid fluid removal during treatment and potential blood loss	Monitor intake and output, weight, blood pressure, pulse, and respirations.	To recognize shifts in fluid balance.
	Monitor blood clotting time.	To monitor effect of anticoagulant therapy.
	Minimize blood loss by careful blood sampling, return of all blood to patient, and pressure applied to fistula puncture sites at end of treatment.	To prevent worsening of anemia that is part of CRF.
	Avoid weight loss greater than 3-4 kg during treatment.	To prevent hypovolemia.
Potential for infection related to invasive procedure and blood transfusion requirements	Identify patient's HBV and HIV status; follow universal precautions for exposure to blood and body fluids.	To protect patient and nurse.
	Use sterile technique to start and stop procedure, for shunt or fistula care; inspect shunt exit sites and fistula needle puncture sites for signs of infection.	To protect patient from potential sources of infection during procedure.
	Monitor temperature, white blood cell count (WBC).	To detect infection; small elevations may reflect significant infections.
	Follow routine testing policies for patients and staff.	To identify change in status.
Altered thought processes related to dialysis disequilibrium syndrome or dialysis dementia	Monitor during and toward end of procedure for headaches, nausea, vomiting, and agitation.	Signs indicating the uneven or too rapid removal of substances occur toward the end of treatment.
	Monitor speech during dialysis; observe for myoclonus and change in behavior.	These signs appear first during hemodialysis.

NURSING DIAGNOSIS	NURSING INTERVENTIONS	RATIONALE
Body image disturbance related to chronic renal failure requiring dependence on a machine	Observe patient's response to chronic illness, altered renal function, other body systems, and possibility of transplantation.	People can vary greatly in their response to such life changes.
	Recognize patient's response to dependence on a machine.	Patient may feel helpless, hopeless; deny reality; personalize the machine; or accept it as necessary.
	Support patient's strengths: self-confidence, determination, and motivation to live.	Dialysis patients are not disabled in all aspects of life.
	Be aware of changes in social involvement; help patient develop or continue interests beyond dialysis and return to as normal a life as possible.	Patient may participate in fewer social-recreational activities, experience life-style changes, and withdraw because of being different.
	Be alert to excessive concerns with losses, depression, self-neglect, noncompliance with medical regimen, and to possibility of suicide; try to keep lines of communication open; encourage questions.	Suicide is possible, and the patient has access to several methods.
	Be aware of effect that loss of libido, impotence, and decreased orgasm has on the patient's marital and sexual life.	To refer patient as appropriate.
	Try to help patient develop realistic expectations of dialysis.	Hemodialysis does not reverse all signs and symptoms of CRF.
Altered family processes related to need for hemodialysis	Recognize the impact CRF with hemodialysis has on the family.	Disruption, expense, and considerable alterations in time commitments may occur.
	Help patient and family recognize demands of illness on family's and patient's need for emotional support. Recognize spouse's fears. Support family's willing cooperation in patient's care and help them to look at ways to reduce domestic tension and unhappiness. Recognize patient's inability to continue family role of homemaker or breadwinner, and help patient accept this through discussion of alternatives. In home dialysis, recognize stresses that family faces and support family in learning about dialysis and carrying out hemodialysis in the home.	Patient outcomes affect the family's ability to cope and vice versa.
Knowledge deficit	See Patient Teaching.	

→ › ›

5 EVALUATE

PATIENT OUTCOME	DATA INDICATING THAT OUTCOME IS REACHED
Weight gain between treatments is in desirable range.	Patient does not gain more than 0.5 kg/day.
Treatments are done safely without hypotension.	Patient does not have hypotension, nausea, or muscle cramps.
No infection develops.	Patient has no signs or symptoms of infection.
Patient's thought processes are normal.	Patient does not develop the signs and symptoms associated with dialysis disequilibrium syndrome or dialysis dementia.
Patient has accepted changes in body image.	Patient and family have adapted to the changes associated with CRF and hemodialysis.
Patient and family have adjusted to life on hemodialysis.	Patient and family have returned to work and social activities as possible; family continues to use health team's support.
Patient and family understand CRF and hemodialysis.	Patient and family can discuss alterations and describe plans for adjusting to them.

PATIENT TEACHING

1. Explain function of normal and artificial kidney.
2. Explain principles of hemodialysis.
3. Explain aseptic technique for needle insertions or shunt care. Explain care of access sites.
4. Teach self-observational skills (temperature, pulse, respirations, blood pressure, intake and output, and weight) and record keeping.
5. Explain components of system with preparation, operation, cleaning, storage (repair and maintenance if home hemodialysis).
6. Explain initiating dialysis, monitoring during dialysis, and discontinuing dialysis.
7. Explain emergencies related to machine and to patient's medical condition.
8. Explain care while off machine: diet, fluid restrictions, medical complications, care of blood access route, medications, and prevention of infection.
9. Explain medical supervision, including help available from medical center, and schedule of return visits, and assistance from the local physician.
10. Review education plan for Chronic Renal Failure (see page 49).

Peritoneal dialysis

Peritoneal dialysis (PD) involves the introduction of dialysate fluid into the abdominal cavity, where the peritoneum acts as a semipermeable membrane between the dialysate and the blood in the abdominal vessels. A machine may be used, or the fluid may be instilled and drained manually from the peritoneal cavity (Figures 11-4 and 11-5).

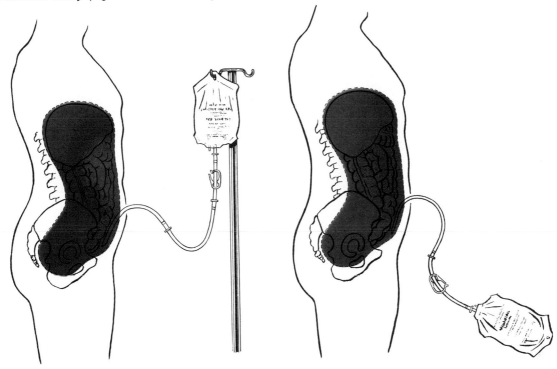

FIGURE 11-4
Peritoneal dialysis. (From Thompson.[27])

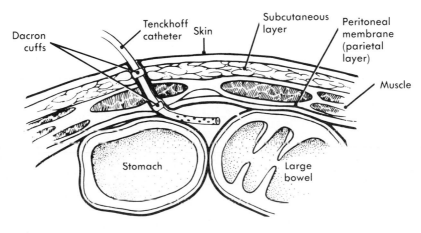

FIGURE 11-5
Peritoneal catheter. (From Lewis and Collier.[15])

Components of peritoneal dialysis solutions include varying amounts of glucose and electrolytes. Glucose at 1.3 mOsm/kg of water yields a 1.5% solution; 2.2 mOsm/kg yields a 4.5% solution; 3.86 mOsm/kg yields a 7% solution. Commonly used concentrations of electrolytes are sodium, 132 mmol/L; potassium, 0 mmol/L; calcium, 1.75 mmol/L; magnesium, 0.5 to 0.75 mmol/L; chloride, 96 mmol/L; and lactate, 35 to 40 mmol/L. The total osmolality is 346 mOsm/kg for the 1.5% solution, 396 mOsm/kg for the 4.5% solution, and 485 mOsm/kg for the 7% solution. The pH of the solution is 5.2. Volumes available range from 250 to 3,000 ml per bag.

Additions may include potassium, 0 to 3 mEq/L, and heparin, 500 to 1,000 U/L.

Continuous ambulatory peritoneal dialysis (CAPD) is an alternative to intermittent peritoneal dialysis for chronic renal failure. A permanent peritoneal dialysis catheter is inserted into the abdomen; a Luer-Lok titanium connector joins the transfer set to the bag of fluid.

CAPD usually involves four exchanges of 1 to 2 L each in 24 hours and dwell times of 4 to 8 hours. Dialysate in plastic bags is used. When the solution is infused, the plastic bag is folded up and concealed under the person's clothes. When the fluid is drained, that bag is discarded and a new bag is attached, and its fluid is instilled for the next cycle. CAPD is self-administered and machine free.

Continuous cycling peritoneal dialysis involves connecting the peritoneal catheter to an automated peritoneal dialysis machine that performs three to seven cycles during the night while the patient sleeps. During the day one cycle of fluid is left in the abdomen. The person is free of dialysis activities during the day, and connections are less frequent than in CAPD.

INDICATIONS

Less rapid treatment needed
Lack of equipment and staff for hemodialysis unavailable
Severe cardiovascular disease
Inadequate access to vascular system
Shock after cardiovascular surgery
Refusal of blood transfusion
Internal hemorrhage or bleeding risk

CONTRAINDICATIONS AND CAUTIONS

Peritonitis
Abdominal adhesions
Recent abdominal surgery

COMPLICATIONS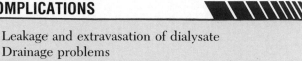

Leakage and extravasation of dialysate
Drainage problems
Hyperglycemia, hypoproteinemia
Weight gain
Infection of catheter exit site or tunnel
Peritonitis (bacterial and nonbacterial)
Bowel adhesions
Respiratory embarrassment

ACCESS DEVICES

Temporary catheter
Permanent catheter
  percutaneous
  subcutaneous

PROCEDURAL GUIDELINES
Before peritoneal dialysis

1. Have patient empty bladder to avoid puncturing it when inserting catheter.
2. Measure and record as baseline data: weight, temperature, pulse, respirations, blood pressure (both lying and standing), abdominal girth.
3. Review blood chemistry values (blood urea nitrogen; serum creatinine, sodium, potassium, and pH; hematocrit). Identify hepatitis B virus (HBV) and human immunodeficiency virus (HIV) status of patient, if known.
4. Use sterile technique as acute peritoneal catheter is placed in abdominal cavity. Permanent catheters are inserted in the operating room. Masks should be worn by patient, nurse, and physician. Use sterile technique during subsequent connections of dialysis fluid to peritoneal catheter and for changing catheter dressings. Observe for infection in catheter insertion site in temporary catheters, and in tunnel site in permanent catheters.
5. After catheter insertion, observe for perforation of bowel (dialysate outflow stained with feces or blood) or bladder (pink or blood-tinged urine).
6. Dry off warmed (37° C [98.6° F]) bottle of fluid before hanging it up, or use plastic bags of solution warmed in folded heating pad on low setting.
7. Add medications to dialysate as ordered. Flush tubing to remove air, and connect to catheter. Anchor connections and tubing securely. Be sure there are no kinks in tubing.

During peritoneal dialysis

1. Measure and record intake, output, weight, temperature, pulse, respirations, and blood pressure regularly. Keep accurate records of dialysis cycles (inflow, dwell, and outflow times). Record strength of solutions used, additions made, and fluid balance (amounts retained or lost).
2. Observe for peritonitis. Collect samples of dialysate for culture and sensitivity tests whenever solution is turbid, bloody, or has an odor, as well as when routinely ordered.
3. Observe for respiratory embarrassment (manifested by dyspnea and rales) resulting from abdomen being too full of fluid or leakage of dialysate into thoracic cavity through a defect in the diaphragm.

Cycle-related problems

Inflow problems. Obstructed catheter (clots, fibrin, omentum, catheter malposition), leakage of fluid around catheter insertion site

Dwell time problems. Prolonged time may cause water depletion or hyperglycemia

Outflow problems. Kinks in tubing or catheter, catheter occluded by loops of bowel, constipation

After peritoneal dialysis

1. Determine fluid balance. Measure weight, temperature, pulse, respirations, blood pressure, and abdominal girth.
2. Check blood chemistries: blood urea nitrogen and serum creatinine, sodium, and potassium.

Care between peritoneal dialysis treatments

1. Encourage adequate protein intake (1.2-5 g/kg/day).
2. Restrict intake of sodium (1,500-2,000 mg/day) and potassium (2,500-3,500 mg/day).
3. Caloric intake, at 35 kcal/kg ideal body weight, should consider the calories from the glucose in the dialysate solution.
4. Fluid restrictions usually range from 0.5 to 1 L/day.
5. Avoid constipation. Consider use of stool softeners and laxatives as needed.
6. Manage continuing uremic problems. (See "Chronic Renal Failure," page 49.)

MEDICAL MANAGEMENT

SURGERY

The peritoneal catheter is inserted into the peritoneal cavity, generally under local anesthetic in the operating room; if the catheter is permanent, it has an internal Dacron cuff that lies between the peritoneum and the abdominal muscles; it has an external cuff that is 1-1.5 cm below the skin at the other end of a 3-4 cm subcutaneous tunnel.

DRUG THERAPY

Anticoagulants: Heparin may be added to dialysate to prevent fibrin formation and obstruction to fluid flow.

Antimicrobials: Used when bacterial peritonitis is diagnosed and often given by both systemic and intraperitoneal routes.

Vitamins (water soluble): To replace those lost in dialysate.

1 ASSESS

ASSESSMENT	OBSERVATIONS
Abdomen	Rigidity, tenderness, cloudy dialysate drainage, decreased or absent bowel sounds; redness, tenderness, and swelling around catheter site
Cardiovascular	Hypervolemia: tachycardia, hypertension, increased central venous pressure, jugular venous distention, extra heart sound (S3), postural edema, weight gain Hypovolemia: hypotension, postural changes, tachycardia, flat neck veins, thirst, dry mucous membranes, weight loss
Neurologic	Headache, lethargy, confusion, coma
Respiratory	Tachypnea, dyspnea, rales, crackles
General	Fever

2 DIAGNOSE

NURSING DIAGNOSIS	SUPPORTIVE ASSESSMENT FINDINGS
Fluid volume excess related to fluid accumulation since last treatment	Weight gain, elevated blood pressure, dyspnea
Fluid volume deficit related to too rapid removal of body fluid during treatment	Lowered blood pressure, nausea, muscle cramps
Potential for infection (peritonitis) related to invasive procedure	Abdominal discomfort, rigidity; rebound tenderness; decreased or absent bowel sounds; cloudy dialysate returns; elevated WBC and positive cultures (serum or dialysate returns); fever; malaise
Altered nutrition: less than body requirements related to protein loss through peritoneum into dialysate and decreased protein intake	Low serum albumin level, weight loss, stomatitis, anorexia, nausea, vomiting
Altered nutrition: potential for more than body requirements related to calorie intake related to glucose in dialysate fluid	Weight gain, signs of hyperglycemia

NURSING DIAGNOSIS	SUPPORTIVE ASSESSMENT FINDINGS
Body image disturbance related to chronic renal failure (CRF) requiring dependence on peritoneal dialysis	Complains of feeling hopeless, helpless; may deny reality or may accept need for dialysis; may have less social activity; may have life-style changes, withdrawal; may have excess concern with losses, depression, self-neglect, noncompliance with regimen, possibility of suicide
Altered family processes related to family member with CRF requiring peritoneal dialysis	Expresses sense of loss, inability to continue usual family roles; spouse or family describes stresses of situation (disruption, expense, altered time commitments); family withdrawal

3 PLAN

Patient goals

1. The patient will avoid the rapid weight gain associated with excess fluid intake.
2. The patient will avoid excess fluid removal during treatment.
3. The patient will not develop peritonitis.
4. The patient will have an adequate protein intake and avoid unwanted weight gain related to excess caloric intake.
5. The patient will accept alterations in body image associated with peritoneal dialysis.
6. The patient and family will discuss changes in the family caused by chronic renal failure requiring peritoneal dialysis and seek help appropriately.
7. The patient and family will understand the purpose of peritoneal dialysis, the process involved, the care required between treatments, and relevant concerns about chronic renal failure. (See "Chronic Renal Failure," page 49.)

4 IMPLEMENT

NURSING DIAGNOSIS	NURSING INTERVENTIONS	RATIONALE
Fluid volume excess related to fluid accumulation since last treatment	Assess weight and blood pressure; monitor laboratory values: blood urea nitrogen; serum creatinine, sodium, potassium, and pH; and hematocrit.	To determine fluid status as basis for treatment parameters. Nitrogenous wastes and electrolytes accumulate between treatment, and anemia is a continuing problem of uremia.
Fluid volume deficit related to too rapid removal of body fluid during treatment	Assess intake and output, weight, blood pressure, pulse, and respirations; avoid excess weight loss (i.e., markedly negative fluid balance as a result of dialysis).	To recognize shifts in fluid balance and to prevent hypovolemia.
Potential for infection related to invasive procedure (peritonitis)	Identify patient's HBV and HIV status, if known; follow universal precautions for exposure to blood and body fluids.	To protect patient and nurse.
	Use sterile technique to start and stop procedure and for access site care.	To protect patient from sources of infection during procedure.

NURSING DIAGNOSIS	NURSING INTERVENTIONS	RATIONALE
	Inspect catheter insertion site for signs of infection; monitor temperature and serum and dialysate WBC.	To detect infection.
Altered nutrition: less than body requirements related to protein loss through peritoneum into dialysate and decreased protein intake	Assess serum protein and glucose and weight.	To determine altered levels.
	Ensure adequate protein intake (see Chronic Renal Failure, page 49).	To replace losses associated with peritoneal dialysis.
Altered nutrition: potential for more than body requirements related to excess calorie intake related to glucose in dialysate fluid	Limit caloric intake in diet and decrease glucose concentration in dialysate fluid or decrease dwell time.	To decrease calories from food or absorbed from dialysate fluid.
Body image disturbance related to chronic renal failure requiring dependence on peritoneal dialysis	Observe patient's response to chronic illness, altered renal function, other body systems, and possibility of transplantation.	People vary greatly in their response to such life changes.
	Recognize patient's response to dependence on peritoneal dialysis; try to keep lines of communication open; encourage questions.	Patient may feel helpless and hopeless, deny reality, personalize the machine, or accept it as necessary.
	Support patient's strengths: self-confidence, determination, and motivation to live.	Dialysis patients are not disabled in all aspects of life.
	Be aware of changes in social involvement; help patient develop or continue interests beyond dialysis and return to as normal a life as possible.	Patient may participate in fewer social-recreational activities, experience life-style changes, and withdraw because of being different.
	Be alert to excessive concerns with losses, depression, self-neglect, noncompliance with medical regimen, and the possibility of suicide.	Suicide is possible, and the patient has access to several methods.
	Be aware of effect of loss of libido, impotence, and decreased orgasm on patient's marital and sexual life.	To refer patient as appropriate.
	Try to help patient develop realistic expectations of dialysis.	Peritoneal dialysis does not reverse all the signs and symptoms of CRF.

NURSING DIAGNOSIS	NURSING INTERVENTIONS	RATIONALE
Altered family processes related to family member with chronic renal failure requiring peritoneal dialysis	Recognize the impact on the family of CRF with peritoneal dialysis.	Disruption, expense, and considerable alterations in time commitments may occur.
	Help patient and family recognize demands of illness on family's and patient's need for emotional support. Recognize family's fears. Support family's willing cooperation in patient's care and help them find ways to reduce domestic tension and unhappiness. Recognize patient's inability to continue family role of homemaker or breadwinner, and help patient accept this through discussion of alternatives. In home peritoneal dialysis, recognize stresses that family faces and support family in learning about dialysis in the home.	Patient outcomes affect the family's ability to cope and vice versa.
Knowledge deficit	See Patient Teaching.	

5 EVALUATE

PATIENT OUTCOME	DATA INDICATING THAT OUTCOME IS REACHED
Weight gain between treatments is in desirable range.	Weight is maintained at or near ideal body weight.
Treatment is done safely without hypotension.	Volume relationships and blood pressure are normal.
Peritonitis is avoided.	No signs or symptoms of peritonitis are present.
Protein and calorie intake meet body requirements.	Serum albumin and glucose levels are within normal limits, and weight is stable.
Patient has accepted changes in body image.	Patient and family have adapted to changes associated with CRF and peritoneal dialysis.
Patient and family have adjusted to life with peritoneal dialysis.	Patient and family have returned to work and social activities as possible. Family and patient continue to use health team's support.
Patient and family understand CRF and peritoneal dialysis.	Patient and family can describe chronic renal failure and medical plan of care. Patient and family describe principles of peritoneal dialysis, plan of care, and correct use of peritoneal dialysis equipment.

PATIENT TEACHING ▪▪▪▪▪▪▪▪▪▪▪▪▪▪▪▪▪▪▪▪▪▪▪▪▪▪▪▪▪▪▪▪▪▪

1. Explain the nature of chronic renal failure.
2. Explain the medical regimen and its rationale, including diet (restricted protein, sodium, and potassium), restricted fluid intake, and medications (purpose, dosage, interval, and adverse reactions).
3. Explain the function of normal and artificial kidneys and the principles of peritoneal dialysis.
4. Teach aseptic technique.
5. Explain components of the system, preparation, operation, cleaning, and storage (repair and maintenance if home dialysis).
6. Explain initiating dialysis, monitoring during dialysis, and discontinuing dialysis.
7. Explain emergencies related to the machine, if used, and to the patient's medical condition.
8. Explain care while off the machine: diet, fluid restrictions, medical complications, care of peritoneal access route, medications, and prevention of infection.
9. Teach self-observational skills (temperature, pulse, respirations, blood pressure, intake and output, and weight) and record keeping.
10. Explain ways to avoid infection.
11. Explain personal hygiene, rest, and exercise.
12. Explain when to call the physician.
13. Explain the plan for medical follow-up.

Continuous Arteriovenous Hemofiltration

Continuous arteriovenous hemofiltration (CAVH) is a process that removes excess water and controls azotemia in patients with uncomplicated acute oliguric renal failure, especially those who are unstable hemodynamically.

CAVH has been especially useful in critical care units. The continuous removal of water allows for less restriction of fluids needed for parenteral nutrition or medications. It is a safe, simple procedure that requires minimum priming volumes (18 to 60 ml). Fluid volumes and electrolyte concentrations change more slowly and thus cause fewer problems. For patients with a hypercatabolic state, hemofiltration can be alternated with hemodialysis to control the more complex azotemia, acid-base abnormalities, electrolyte excesses, and anemia, thus limiting the number of conventional hemodialysis treatments needed.

Using a highly permeable, hollow fiber filter such as the Amicon Diafilter 20, plasma water and all unbound substances with molecular weights between 500 and 10,000 daltons can move from the vascular space and through the membrane of the fiber to form an ultrafiltrate (Figure 11-6).

Arterial and venous access sites are needed. The blood is propelled by the force of arterial blood pressure through an extracorporeal circuit, which includes the hemofilter, and back to the patient. The tubing is kept as short as possible to decrease resistance to flow in the system. For the process to work successfully, the mean arterial pressure (MAP) must be 60 mm Hg, and the hematocrit must be less than 40%. The filter has a large surface area, a high sieving coefficient, and low resistance so it can be used in patients with low mean arterial pressures. Since the volume in the circuit is small, unstable patients can tolerate CAVH treatments. Percutaneous cannulation of the femoral artery and vein is frequently used for access, but an arteriovenous shunt may be used.

Blood leaves the arterial cannula and enters the tubing leading to the hemofilter. A continuous infusion of heparin is added to the blood before it enters the hemofilter to prevent clotting. The pressure difference in the hemofilter (arterial pressure minus the oncotic pressure and the low pressure on the outer side of the hollow fibers) allows water and solutes to cross the membrane, forming an ultrafiltrate. The process is similar to the filtration process of the glomerular basement membrane in the kidney. The resulting ultrafiltrate is composed of water and solutes (sodium, potassium, chloride urea, glucose, creatinine, uric acid, and phosphate); it drains into a collection device. The level of the collection device is important in determining the rate of ultrafiltration. Raising the level decreases the negative pressure and thus the rate of ultrafiltration, whereas lowering it increases the negative pressure and the rate of ultrafiltration. Generally, with adequate blood flow rates (30 to 120 ml/minute), the ultrafiltration rate is 5 to 16 ml/minute or 7 to 24 L/24 hours. As the blood leaves the hemofilter, it is rediluted with solutions that provide the water, electrolytes, and nutrition needed by the patient. Unwanted electrolytes are not replaced, and thus the patient's serum levels decline.

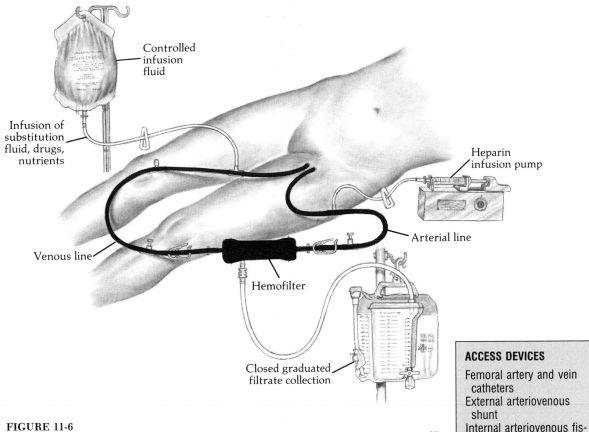

FIGURE 11-6
Continuous arteriovenous hemofiltration with femoral cannulation. (From Thompson.[27])

> **ACCESS DEVICES**
>
> Femoral artery and vein catheters
> External arteriovenous shunt
> Internal arteriovenous fistula

INDICATIONS

Overhydration in patients who are unresponsive to diuretics, who have cardiovascular instability or severe coagulopathies, or who need parenteral nutrition

Elderly patient with serious cerebrovascular disease, coronary artery sclerosis, or uncomplicated acute renal failure

Acute renal failure with multiple organ system failure

Inability to tolerate conventional hemodialysis or peritoneal dialysis

CONTRAINDICATIONS

Hypercatabolic state
Hyperkalemia
Poisoning
Low blood flow states (MAP <60 mm Hg)
Shock or low colloid oncotic pressure
Congestive heart failure
Severe atherosclerosis

COMPLICATIONS

Clotting in filter or tubing
Access problems (bleeding, clotting, infection)
Excessive fluid removal

PROCEDURAL GUIDELINES
Preparation for CAVH

1. Assemble equipment; prime hemofilter circuit. With new filters, rinse well to remove glycerin coating, ethylene oxide used in sterilization, and all air bubbles.
2. Measure and record for baseline data: weight, blood pressure, temperature, pulse, respirations, central venous pressure, pulmonary artery pressures, and cardiac output, as appropriate.

3. Review pretreatment laboratory values: blood urea nitrogen; serum creatinine, sodium, potassium, calcium, magnesium, and phosphate; WBC, hemoglobin, and hematocrit; activated clotting time, prothrombin time, partial thromboplastin time, and platelet count. Note patient's HBV and HIV status, if known.

4. Assist with insertion of catheters or connection to existing access device using sterile technique. Begin anticoagulation, if ordered. Connect infusion line for the replacement fluid ordered.

During CAVH

1. Open arterial and venous lines and inspect filter, tubing, and connections (taping all without screw locks). Secure hemofilter to patient to prevent inadvertent dislodgement. Open ultrafiltration port, and begin infusion of replacement fluid. Begin heparin infusion.

2. Monitor patient: direct arterial pressure and other hemodynamic parameters if available; pulses distal to catheters; activated clotting time. Assess for bleeding. Regulate heparin infusion. Keep blood and drainage lines visible.

3. Monitor and regulate ultrafiltration rate. Measure other sources of output. Regulate fluid replacement and measure all sources of input. Calculate balance hourly and adjust rates as indicated.

Termination of CAVH

1. Close ultrafiltrate port. Discontinue infusions of replacement fluid and heparin.

2. Clamp arterial and then venous lines. Remove acute catheters, and apply prolonged pressure to sites. Provide routine care to shunt or fistula, if used.

MEDICAL MANAGEMENT

GENERAL MANAGEMENT

A portion of the fluid removed and discarded is replaced with water and solutes needed by the patient; typical replacement fluid contains sodium (140 mEq/L); potassium (0-2 mEq/L); acetate (35-40 mEq/L); magnesium (1.5 mEq/L); calcium (3.5 mEq/L); chloride (110-120 mEq/L); and dextrose (0-200 mg/dl); infusion rates range from 400-600 ml/h.

Nutritional needs can be met without fluid overload by infusing parenteral nutrition solutions with the replacement fluids.

DRUG THERAPY

Anticoagulant agents: Heparin sodium: initial dose 500-2500 USP U; continuous infusion 500 USP U/h if no coagulation abnormalities; keep clotting time between 15 and 30 min; check prothrombin time and partial thromboplastin time as ordered.

---

1   ASSESS

ASSESSMENT	OBSERVATIONS
Cardiovascular	Hypervolemia: tachycardia, hypertension, increased central venous pressure, jugular venous distention, extra heart sounds (S3), lung sounds (crackles), postural edema, weight gain
	Hypovolemia: hypotension, postural changes, tachycardia, flat neck veins, thirst, dry mucous membranes, weight loss
	Vascular access site: bleeding, red, swollen, tender

2 DIAGNOSE

NURSING DIAGNOSIS	SUPPORTIVE ASSESSMENT FINDINGS
Fluid volume excess related to fluid accumulation due to altered renal function or too rapid infusion of replacement fluid	Dyspnea, tachycardia, extra heart sound (S3), lung crackles, jugular venous distention, edema, weight gain; increased central venous pressure, arterial pressure, pulmonary artery pressures
Potential fluid volume deficit related to too rapid removal of fluid (ultrafiltration) due to excess negative pressure or inadequate fluid replacement	Thirst, dry mucous membranes, flat neck veins, tachycardia, hypotension, postural changes; decreased central venous pressure or cardiac output, pulmonary artery pressures; weight loss
Potential for infection related to invasive procedure	Skin broken at access site
Impaired physical mobility related to presence of access device and connections to hemofilter	Limited range of motion in extremity adjacent to access site; bed rest

3 PLAN

Patient goals

1. The patient will demonstrate normal fluid balance.
2. The patient will not develop an infection.
3. The patient will not develop complications of immobility.
4. The patient and family will understand the purpose of continuous arteriovenous hemofiltration.

4 IMPLEMENT

NURSING DIAGNOSIS	NURSING INTERVENTIONS	RATIONALE
Fluid volume excess related to fluid accumulation due to altered renal function or too rapid infusion of replacement fluid	Assess weight, blood pressure, pulse, respirations, and intake and output.	To determine fluid status.
	Monitor laboratory values: blood urea nitrogen; serum creatinine, sodium, potassium, calcium, magnesium, and phosphate; hemoglobin and hematocrit; and clotting time.	To determine electrolyte balance, accumulation of nitrogenous wastes, effects of solute removal, and extent of anemia related to renal failure.

NURSING DIAGNOSIS	NURSING INTERVENTIONS	RATIONALE
	Monitor rate of ultrafiltration.	A 20% decrease in rate may mean a clotted hemofilter.
	Observe color of blood in hemofilter, color of ultrafiltrate collected, and whether air bubbles are present.	Darkening of blood in the circuit or streaks in the filter means clotting in the filter; pink or red in the ultrafiltrate means leaks or rupture in the hemofilter; air bubbles mean air is entering the system, disconnected lines, excess negative pressure, or leaks or cracks in the hemofilter.
Potential fluid volume deficit related to too rapid removal of fluid (ultrafiltration) due to excess negative pressure or inadequate fluid replacement	Assess hourly intake and output, weight, blood pressure, pulse, and respirations; note rate of ultrafiltration.	To recognize shifts in fluid balance and prevent hypovolemia.
	Control level of ultrafiltrate collection device.	Distance below hemofilter controls amount of negative pressure and rate of fluid removal.
Potential for infection related to invasive procedure	Identify patient's HBV and HIV status, if known; follow universal precautions for exposure to blood or body fluids.	To protect patient and nurse.
	Use sterile technique to start and stop procedure and to care for access device site.	To protect patient from potential sources of infection during procedure.
	Inspect site for redness, swelling, tenderness, and drainage; monitor temperature and WBC.	To detect infection.
Impaired physical mobility related to presence of access device and connections to hemofilter	Do range-of-motion exercises to other extremities; have patient deep breathe, turn, and cough regularly; perform skin care.	To prevent complications of bed rest.

5 EVALUATE

PATIENT OUTCOME	DATA INDICATING THAT OUTCOME IS REACHED
Fluid balance within normal limits.	Absence of signs and symptoms of fluid overload or dehydration.
No infection is present.	Temperature normal, white blood cell count normal, no signs of infection at access site.
Patient has no complications of immobility.	No pneumonia, deep vein thrombosis, skin breakdown, decreased range of motion.
Patient and family understand hemofiltration.	Patient and family understand procedure.

PATIENT TEACHING

1. Explain the purpose of hemofiltration, the equipment, and its role in life support.

2. Explain the reasons for bed rest.

Renal Transplantation

Renal transplantation (RT) is the surgical insertion of a human kidney from a living donor or a cadaver into a patient with end-stage renal disease, thus replacing the lost renal function. A donor is sought when the patient's serum creatinine is around 5 mg/dl, serum blood urea nitrogen is greater than 70 mg/dl, and creatinine clearance is 15 ml/minute. When successful, a transplant restores the recipient to a healthy, useful life. If a transplant is unsuccessful, the patient can return to dialysis or have a second transplant.

The number of kidney transplants has increased each year since 1978. In 1988, 8,932 transplantations were performed; 6,651 of these transplants came from cadavers and 1,599 from living donors related to the recipient. Patient survival and graft function has improved since 1983 when cyclosporine was introduced. By the end of 1988 there were 36,976 patients with end-stage renal disease who had functioning transplanted kidneys.[28]

The donated kidney is placed in the retroperitoneal area in the iliac fossa on the contralateral side. Thus a donated left kidney is placed in the recipient's right iliac fossa (Figure 11-7). The donor's artery is anastomosed end to end to the recipient's hypogastric artery.

The donor's vein is anastomosed to the recipient's internal iliac vein. The donor's ureter is implanted in the recipient's bladder.

The kidney from a living related donor is flushed with a cold solution and then placed in the recipient. A cadaveric kidney may be preserved by flushing followed by cold storage or by constant perfusion with a special solution.

Transplantation is usually the treatment of choice in children. Aging patients may have problems with trans-

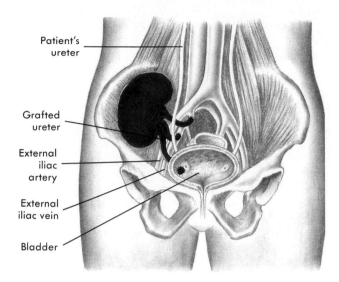

FIGURE 11-7
Renal transplant. (From Thompson.[27])

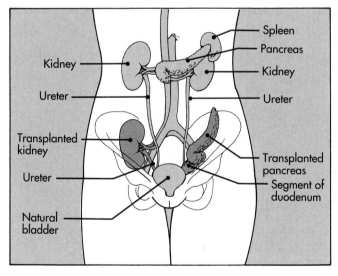

FIGURE 11-8
Transplanted kidney and pancreas.

plantation because of atherosclerosis or other serious systemic disorders. Patients with diabetes are increasingly considered for transplantation, but the problems with the continuing diabetic condition increase complications such as infection. The use of corticosteroids exacerbates problems in glucose level control. Combined pancreas and kidney transplants are being used for diabetic patients (Figure 11-8).

INDICATIONS

End-stage renal disease
Loss of solitary kidney through trauma
Inability to adjust to dialysis

CONTRAINDICATIONS AND CAUTIONS

Age under 5 years or older than 50 years
Malignancy
Acute uncontrollable infection
Hepatic disease
Presence of antikidney antibodies
Severe psychosis
Tuberculosis or peptic ulcer disease
Chronic respiratory insufficiency
Severe atherosclerosis
Severe myocardial dysfunction

COMPLICATIONS

Acute tubular necrosis
Spontaneous rupture of graft
Organ rejection
Ureteral fistula or obstruction
Perirenal hematoma, lymphocele, or abscess
Renal artery stenosis or thrombosis
Renal vein thrombosis
Infection
Reappearance of primary renal disease

PROCEDURAL GUIDELINES

Before transplantation

1. Assess patient's preoperative status.
2. Teach patient and family what to expect during surgery and in the early postoperative period. (Refer to pages 189 to 191.)

After transplantation

1. Assess vital signs and urine output every 15 minutes, gradually lengthening interval. Urine begins to flow in 2 to 10 minutes after revascularization at 5 to 10 ml/minute. Careful fluid replacement prevents overhydration or underhydration.

2. Keep patient flat (head of bed may be elevated to 30 degrees) with legs straight to prevent tension on the anastomoses; turn only to operative side; may ambulate within 24 hours but should not sit.
3. Anchor catheters; do not clamp them, but connect to a closed drainage system.
4. Measure urethral and ureteral volumes and record. Urine may be bloody at first. Cessation of urine may be caused by a clot, and irrigation of the urethral catheter may be needed to dislodge it. If ureteral catheter needs irrigating, extreme care is required to avoid damage to the ureteral anastomosis.
5. Try to maintain patency of blood access device in case dialysis is required in the immediate postoperative period.

CRITERIA FOR KIDNEY TRANSPLANTATION

Criteria for recipient
End-stage renal disease
Age 5 to 50 years
No uncorrectable abnormalities of other major body systems such as infection (HBV or HIV), urologic problems, severe cardiac disease, chronic pulmonary disease, preexisting cancer, or psychiatric disorder

Criteria for living related donor
Age 18 to 55 years
Excellent physical and mental health
Immunologically compatible with recipient

Criteria for cadaveric donor
Age 4 to 55 years
Normal renal function tests
No HBV or HIV infection
Immunologically compatible with recipient
No systemic disease such as infection, cancer, or advanced cardiovascular disease, including hypertension or renal-urologic disorders
No hypoxia or hypotension before death

SELECTED SIDE EFFECTS OF MAJOR IMMUNOSUPPRESSIVE DRUGS

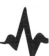

Drug	Side Effects
Cyclosporine (Sandimmune)	Renal and hepatic toxicity, hypertension, hirsutism, gingival hyperplasia, nausea, vomiting, diarrhea
Azathioprine (Imuran)	Nausea, vomiting, leukopenia, anemia, thrombocytopenia, hepatic toxicity
Prednisone	Depression, euphoria, hypertension, decreased wound healing, petechiae, ecchymoses, hirsutism, acne, adrenal suppression, muscle wasting, osteoporosis, redistribution of fat (moon face, buffalo hump)
Muromonab-CD3 (Orthoclone OKT 3)	Fever, chills, nausea, vomiting, diarrhea, chest tightness, dyspnea, pulmonary edema

MEDICAL MANAGEMENT

GENERAL MANAGEMENT

Dialysis may be needed.

Fluid intake should balance output: about 400-600 ml (about the amount of insensible losses) plus amount equal to 24-h urine volume; patient should avoid dehydration and volume excess.

Nutritional modifications to achieve or maintain adequate nutritional status and to reduce work of diseased kidney.

No dietary restrictions after gastrointestinal function returns; caloric intake may need to be restricted if appetite is increased by corticosteroids; if renal function is decreased or hypertension continues, patient may need to restrict protein, sodium, and potassium and increase calories supplied by fats and carbohydrates.

Routine cultures of likely places for infection (urinary tract, wound, throat, and blood) may be done, since the immunosuppressive agents used after transplantation mask the signs and symptoms of infection. All immunosuppressive agents currently in use affect phagocytosis, cellular immunity, or humoral immunity. Liver function is monitored because azathioprine can cause cholestatic hepatitis. Cyclosporine may damage the kidney and liver. Muromonab-CD3 causes a flulike symptom complex.

The signs and symptoms of rejection are monitored. If rejection occurs and is not reversed, the graft is removed and the patient is returned to dialysis. The most frequent complications are related to technical problems, the effects of preexisting uremia, graft rejection, and the side effects of immunosuppression.

DRUG THERAPY

Immunosuppressive agents: Cyclosporine (Cyclosporin A), azathioprine (Imuran), antilymphocyte globulin, antithymocyte globulin (ATG), cyclophosphamide (Cytoxan), prednisone.

Antacids: With prednisone, aluminum carbonate or phosphate.

Insulin preparations: For hyperglycemia associated with prednisone therapy, highly individualized.

Antirejection drugs: Methylprednisolone in high doses (1 g/day for 3 days), Muromonab-CD3 (Orthoclone OKT3) for 10-14 days

1 ASSESS

ASSESSMENT	OBSERVATIONS
Renal	Rejection: decreased urine production and creatinine clearance; increased serum creatinine and blood urea nitrogen; proteinuria, decreased urinary sodium, urea, and creatinine; tenderness over graft; decreased renal blood flow and increased size of graft by renal scan; fever, weight gain, and hypertension; anxiety, apathy, and lethargy
Urinary tract	Bacteriuria, pyuria, cloudy and foul-smelling urine

2 DIAGNOSE

NURSING DIAGNOSIS	SUPPORTIVE ASSESSMENT FINDINGS
Potential fluid volume excess or deficit related to postoperative diuresis, altered renal perfusion (acute tubular necrosis, rejection)	Altered pulse, respirations, blood pressure, central venous pressure, weight, intake, output, and blood chemistries
Pain related to surgery: incision, bladder spasms	Incisional discomfort on moving; lower abdominal discomfort, guarding behavior
Potential for infection related to immunosuppression, surgery, catheters in urinary tract	Fever, leukocytosis, any other signs or symptoms of infection, wound changes (red, swollen, draining), cloudy and foul-smelling urine
Body image disturbance related to need to accept a new body part	Patient expresses guilt, concern for donor
Altered family processes related to change in patient's condition	Family expresses concern about what to expect of patient after surgery

3 PLAN

Patient goals

1. The patient will demonstrate normal fluid balance.
2. The patient will be free of pain.
3. The patient will not develop an infection.
4. The patient will adjust to altered body image associated with acquisition of a new kidney.
5. The patient and family will adjust to alterations in the family associated with change in the patient's condition.
6. The patient and family will be knowledgeable about home care and will understand follow-up instructions.

➔ ❯ ❯

4   IMPLEMENT

NURSING DIAGNOSIS	NURSING INTERVENTIONS	RATIONALE
Potential fluid volume excess or deficit related to postoperative diuresis, altered renal perfusion (acute tubular necrosis, rejection)	Assess blood pressure, pulse, respirations, breath sounds, central venous pressure, cardiac output, intake and output, and weight.	To determine fluid status; patient is sensitive to changes in fluid volumes.
	Monitor laboratory values: blood urea nitrogen; serum creatinine, uric acid, sodium, potassium, calcium, magnesium, and phosphate; hematocrit and hemoglobin; urine levels of creatinine, urea, uric acid, sodium, potassium, blood, and protein.	To assess functioning of new kidney.
	Balance fluid intake with output.	To avoid hypervolemia or hypovolemia.
	Monitor dialysis access device; no blood pressure readings or venipunctures should be done on that arm.	Dialysis may be needed in the postoperative period.
Pain related to surgery: incision, bladder spasms	Assess need for analgesic drugs. Administer as ordered, and monitor response.	To control surgical pain.
	When catheter is out, encourage patient to void frequently to avoid overdistention of bladder.	Unused bladder may spasm as it fills with urine.
Potential for infection related to immunosuppression, surgery, catheters in urinary tract	Use sterile technique for wound and catheter care.	To protect patient with increased susceptibility to infection because of antirejection drugs.
	Inspect incision.	To detect changes early; little drainage is expected.
	Monitor temperature. Monitor laboratory values: serum WBC, urine for bacteria, pyuria, cloudy appearance, cultures.	Signs and symptoms of infection may be masked by immunosuppression, so even minor increases are important.
	Monitor visitors.	To avoid exposure to individuals with infections.
	Encourage deep breathing, coughing, turning, and early ambulation.	To prevent respiratory complications.
Body image disturbance related to need to accept a new body part	Be aware that patient may feel both guilty and concerned about the donor.	Mixed feelings are not unexpected.
	Side effects of immunosuppressive drugs may change appearance.	Obvious changes may include alopecia, hirsutism, redistribution of body fat, and acne. (See page 159 for side effects.)

NURSING DIAGNOSIS	NURSING INTERVENTIONS	RATIONALE
Altered family processes related to change in patient's condition	Keep lines of communication open; assist in patient-family communication.	Family is used to a chronically ill person; a return to health may require changes in family patterns. The patient may be perceived as too independent or not independent enough.
	Recognize the feelings of the living related donor.	Before the transplant the donor may have felt like a hero or heroine; after surgery, all the attention may focus on the recipient.
	Inform the family of changes that are possible when taking immunosuppressive drugs, especially prednisone.	Emotional as well as physical changes may occur.
	Discuss the possible need for contraception, if appropriate.	Potency may return in males; ovulation, menses, and libido may return in females.
	If patient and family do not already know others who have gone through this situation, offer to introduce them to a patient and family.	Family-to-family assistance is often useful.
	Refer family to other professional colleagues (social workers, psychologists) if they can better meet family's needs (financial concerns, occupational problems, and the need for family counseling beyond nurse's expertise).	Professional colleagues often can be helpful in meeting family needs.
Knowledge deficit	See Patient Teaching.	

5 EVALUATE

PATIENT OUTCOME	DATA INDICATING THAT OUTCOME IS REACHED
Fluid balance is within normal limits.	No signs or symptoms of fluid overload or dehydration are noted; renal function tests are within normal limits.
Patient is free of pain.	Patient does not complain of pain.
Patient is free of infection.	Patient has no signs or symptoms of infection in incision or urine or elsewhere.
Patient has accepted changes in body image.	Patient and family have adapted to changes associated with transplantation and immunosuppression.

→ > >

PATIENT OUTCOME	DATA INDICATING THAT OUTCOME IS REACHED
Patient and family have adjusted to life after transplantation.	Patient and family have returned to work and social activities.
Patient and family are knowledgeable about patient's condition.	Patient and family demonstrate knowledge of home care and follow-up care.

PATIENT TEACHING

1. Preparation for discharge includes teaching the following:
   a. Self-observational skills (temperature, pulse, respiration, weight, intake and output, urine collection, and record keeping)
   b. Medications: name, dosage, strength, schedule, purpose, and side effects
   c. Diet: restriction, if any (patient should avoid becoming overweight)
   d. Fluids: restriction, if any
   e. Signs and symptoms of rejection and infection
   f. Important laboratory values (serum creatinine, blood urea nitrogen level, white blood cell count, calcium, and phosphate); with an arteriovenous fistula, do not have blood pressure taken or blood drawn in that arm

2. Long-term follow-up includes teaching the following:
   a. Medical appointment schedule for routine follow-up; plans for telephone communication between appointments
   b. Personal hygiene, prevention of infection, care of minor trauma, contraceptive device, and need for regular dental and eye examinations
   c. Body changes resulting from uremia and long-term anti-rejection therapy, including increased possibility of malignancies
   d. Physical activity levels (daily exercise, avoidance of contact sports, and avoidance of seat belts across the hips) and return to work and other activities
   e. Resources for rehabilitation (including vocational)

Kidney Surgery

Kidney surgery can be an open or closed (percutaneous) procedure. Open surgery of the kidney is done to obtain biopsy specimens, remove all or part of a kidney, repair traumatic injuries, or implant a donated organ. Percutaneous procedures are used for removing renal calculi and establishing urinary drainage.

Open renal biopsy is used to obtain a specimen if the percutaneous approach is not successful or if a person has a single kidney or severe hypertension or coagulopathy. (See "Kidney Biopsy," page 35.)

Nephrectomy is the surgical removal of the whole kidney or part of it (see Figures 11-9 and 11-10). A partial nephrectomy usually involves the upper or lower poles of the kidney, since they have well-defined blood supplies. In a simple nephrectomy, the kidney is removed but not the adrenal gland, surrounding fat, or fascia. A radical nephrectomy is the removal of the kidney, adrenal gland, perirenal fat, upper ureter, and Gerota's fascia.

Nephrolithotomy is the removal of a calculus through an opening in the renal parenchyma.

Pyelolithotomy is the removal of a calculus through an opening in the renal pelvis.

Pyeloplasty is the procedure used to repair the renal pelvis (e.g., after hydronephrosis).

Nephrostomy (open) is the creation of an opening into the kidney to provide temporary or permanent drainage when a retrograde catheter is not possible (Figure 11-11). An incision is made into the renal pelvis and out through the renal parenchyma to place a catheter that will drain the renal pelvis. The catheter is anchored in the renal pelvis, and the pelvis is sutured. The distal end of the catheter extends through the kidney and exits the skin through a stab incision in the flank.

Percutaneous nephrostomy is the insertion of a catheter through the skin into the renal pelvis to establish temporary or permanent urinary drainage (Figure 11-12).

Renal transplantation. See page 158.

Percutaneous nephrolithotomy is the use of a rigid or flexible nephroscope (under general anesthesia and x-ray guidance) to make a tract through the skin and other tissues to the kidney (Figure 11-13). Instruments such as a stone basket, stone grasper, or a lithotriptor probe (percutaneous lithotripsy) may be used to remove stones or break them up before removal.

Flank approach

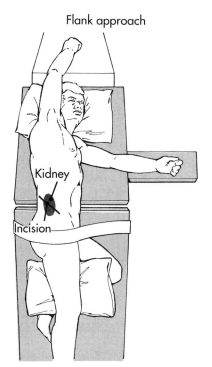

Lumbar approach

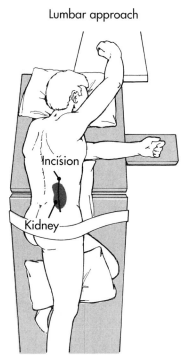

Thoracoabdominal approach

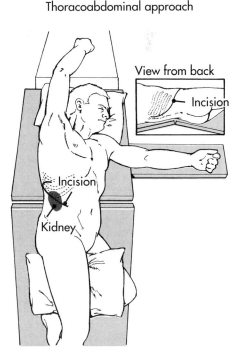

FIGURE 11-9
Types of incisions for kidney surgery.

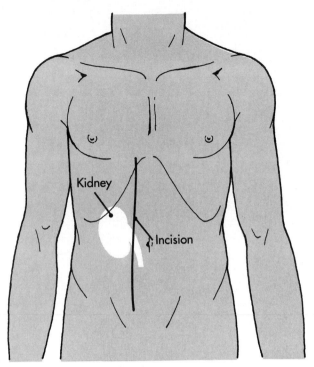
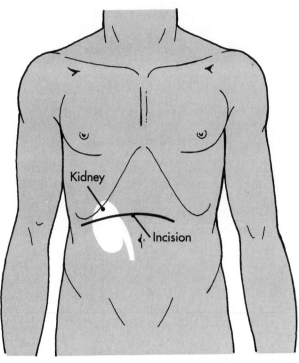

Vertical incision   Horizontal incision

FIGURE 11-10
Abdominal approaches to kidney surgery.

TYPES OF INCISIONS USED
Flank
Subcostal
Transcostal and intercostal
Lumbar
Abdominal
Subcostal
Thoracolumbar
The type of incision used depends on the site of the defect. The approach may be retroperitoneal or transperitoneal.

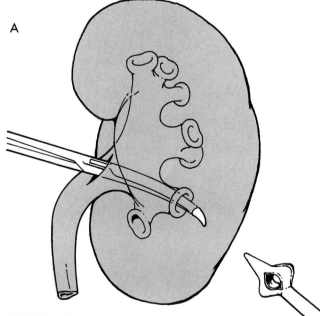

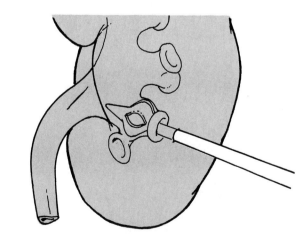

FIGURE 11-11
Open nephrostomy. **A,** Tube brought through renal capsule. **B,** Tube in renal pelvis.

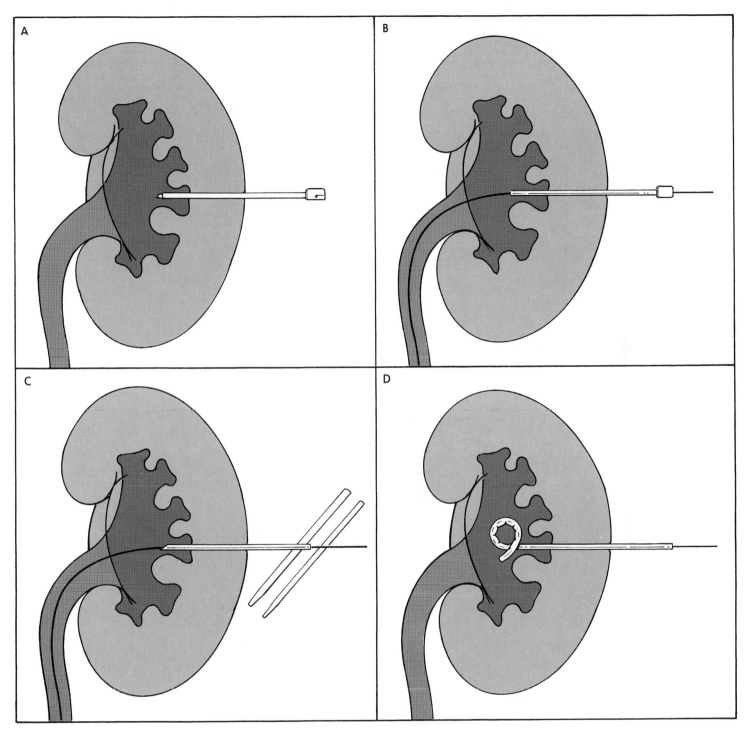

FIGURE 11-12
Percutaneous nephrostomy. **A,** Needle with obturator. **B,** Guidewire in place. **C,** Tract is dilated. **D,** Drainage catheter.

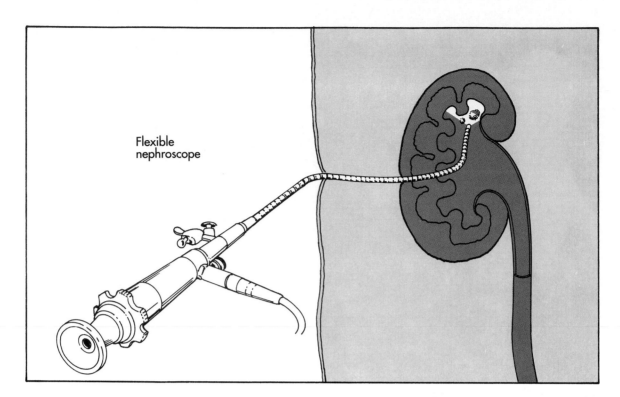

Flexible
nephroscope

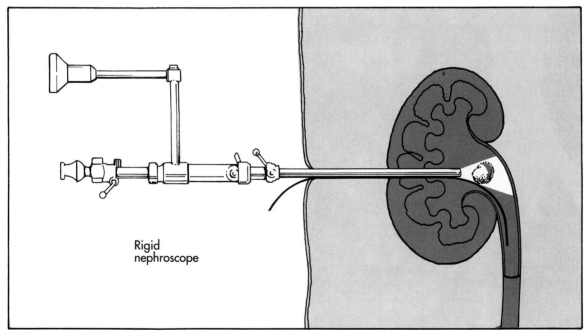

Rigid
nephroscope

FIGURE 11-13
Flexible and rigid nephroscopes.

PROCEDURAL GUIDELINES

1. Prepare the patient and family for the surgical procedure planned and the care that will follow it. Discuss the location of the incision, tubes, stents, drains, and so forth; routines for deep breathing, coughing, turning; pain relief.
2. Determine functional level of each kidney. Treat any urinary tract infection. Bacteriuria impairs healing; leakage of infected urine into soft tissues may cause abscesses; obstruction may cause acute bacterial nephritis.
3. Prepare the patient for surgery: bowel and skin preparation as ordered. Preoperative sedation is used.

INDICATIONS

Staghorn calculus
Hemorrhage
Hydronephrosis
Renovascular hypertension
Neoplasms
Renal donation
Trauma
Vascular disease

CONTRAINDICATIONS AND CAUTIONS

Nephrectomy
  Bilateral disease
  Single kidney
Percutaneous renal procedures
  Septicemia
  Urinary tract obstruction

COMPLICATIONS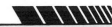

Nephrectomy
  Hemorrhage
  Infection
  Pneumothorax
Percutaneous renal procedures
  Hemorrhage
  Infection
  Urinary extravasation
  Perirenal hematoma

Caution is necessary before removing a diseased kidney (even if the other one is normal) if the disorder is likely to affect the remaining kidney in the future (urolithiasis, renal vascular disease, infection, inflammatory processes).

1 ASSESS

ASSESSMENT	OBSERVATIONS
General	Fever, incisional pain
Skin (incision)	Redness, swelling, drainage of urine, blood
Urinary tract	Urine output from each tube or catheter (amount, character); bleeding; absence of urine

2 DIAGNOSE

NURSING DIAGNOSIS	SUPPORTIVE ASSESSMENT FINDINGS
Impaired skin integrity related to surgical incision	Surgical incision present
Potential fluid volume deficit related to decreased intake by mouth, increased losses due to diuresis, hemorrhage	Nothing by mouth after midnight before surgery and in immediate postoperative period; output greater than intravenous intake; excessive blood loss through tubes, catheters

→ > >

NURSING DIAGNOSIS	SUPPORTIVE ASSESSMENT FINDINGS
Pain related to surgical incision	Pain, guarding behavior noted
Altered patterns of urinary elimination related to use of tubes, catheters, drains	Urethral and ureteral catheters, ureteral stent, nephrostomy tube, Penrose drains may be in place
Potential for infection related to break in skin barrier and presence of catheters	Fever; increased WBC; red, swollen incision; purulent drainage; pyuria, bacteriuria

3 PLAN

Patient goals

1. The patient will regain skin integrity.
2. The patient will have normal fluid balance.
3. The patient will be free of pain.
4. The patient will be free of infection.

5. The patient will return to normal urinary elimination.
6. The patient will be knowledgeable about the condition requiring surgery, home care, and necessary follow-up medical care.

4 IMPLEMENT

NURSING DIAGNOSIS	NURSING INTERVENTIONS	RATIONALE
Impaired skin integrity related to surgical incision	After surgery, assess incision site for signs of bleeding and infection.	To detect complications promptly.
	Note amount and kinds of drainage through tubes and drains.	Urine leakage is expected for several days with incisions into the kidney.
	Keep area clean and dry.	To prevent skin breakdown and promote healing.
Potential fluid volume deficit related to decreased intake by mouth, increased losses due to diuresis, hemorrhage	Measure intake and output and weight every 24 h. Assess vital signs, hemoglobin, and hematocrit.	To identify alterations in fluid status promptly.
Pain related to surgical incision	Assess need for analgesic drugs; administer drug as ordered; record response.	To determine need for drug and relieve pain; to determine the effectiveness of timing and dosage; to identify side effects.

NURSING DIAGNOSIS	NURSING INTERVENTIONS	RATIONALE
Altered patterns of urinary elimination related to use of tubes, catheters, drains	Keep any drainage tubes patent, unkinked, and anchored.	To maintain urine flow and avoid inadvertent displacement.
	Monitor amount of urine from each tube.	To ensure adequate drainage and avoid tension on the suture line and to promote healing. Tubes may include a stent (a catheter inserted in the ureter), a nephrostomy tube, an incisional drain, and a urethral catheter. Drainage may continue for several days after incision into kidney; hematuria can be expected for 12-24 hr.
Potential for infection related to break in skin barrier and presence of catheters	Assess temperature, WBC, wound drainage, and urine for pyuria and bacteriuria.	To detect any infection promptly.
Knowledge deficit	See Patient Teaching.	

5 EVALUATE

PATIENT OUTCOME	DATA INDICATING THAT OUTCOME IS REACHED
Skin integrity is unimpaired.	Incision has healed.
Fluid balance is within normal limits.	Fluid intake is adequate and balances output.
Patient has no pain.	Patient does not complain of pain.
Urinary elimination pattern is normal.	All tubes, drains, and catheters have been removed.
No infection is present.	Patient has no fever and has normal WBC and urinalysis.
Patient and family are knowledgeable about the condition requiring surgery.	Patient and family understand the kidney problem, home care, and needed follow-up medical care.

PATIENT TEACHING

1. Explain the cause of the problem requiring surgery.
2. Explain home care of the incision, drains, or tubes as needed.
3. Teach techniques for preventing recurrence of renal problem.
4. Explain any need for follow-up medical care.

RENAL TRAUMA

Even though the kidneys are well-protected by their location, they may be injured. The kidney is the most frequently injured organ of the urinary tract. Kidney injuries are caused by blunt and penetrating forces. Blunt trauma causes most renal injuries (80-85%). Frequently there are associated injuries that are serious. Fractures of the vertebral processes or the 11th or 12th rib are common causes of lacerations. Kidneys with preexisting abnormalities such as tumors, hydronephrosis, or congenital anomalies are particularly at risk.

Causes of renal injuries

Motor vehicle accidents
Pedestrian accidents
Fights, assaults
Falls
Contact sports
Occupational injuries

Mechanisms of injury

Blunt force
    Sharp blow to abdomen, flank, back, lower chest
    Compression (crushing)
    Acceleration-deceleration
Penetrating force
    Knives, bullets, flying projectiles

Severity of injury

Minor: bruising, superficial lacerations, subcapsular hematoma
Major: deep lacerations, loss of kidney integrity
Critical: damage to renal artery or vein, shattered kidney with multiple lacerations and fragments

Classification of injuries

Contusion: bruises or minor tears without tears in the capsule
Laceration: tears in renal parenchyma with damage to capsule or calyces or both
Fragmentation: multiple deep lacerations with rupture or shattering of kidney
Major renal vessel injury: damage to renal artery or vein; complete or partial avulsion, stretch injury of renal artery resulting in intimal tears and thrombosis

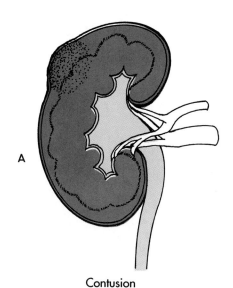

Contusion

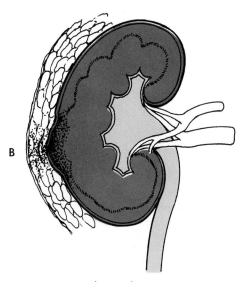

Laceration

Various types of renal trauma. **A,** Contusion. **B,** Laceration. **C,** Fragmentation. **D,** Major vascular injury.

ASSESSMENT

Signs and symptoms vary with type of injury and whether other abdominal organs are injured. First complete the primary survey, ensuring airway, breathing, circulation, and safety of cervical spine. In the secondary survey assess the potential for renal injury. Observe for ecchymosis on flank or abdomen; flank tenderness or pain. Pain may be caused by increased renal capsular tension (dull ache), clots in the ureter (renal colic), or retroperitoneal hematoma (diffuse abdominal pain). Feel for expanding mass in flank or abdomen. Observe for hematuria and altered urine output.

Useful diagnostic studies include:

Kidney-ureter-bladder (KUB) x-ray	Renal arteriogram
Intravenous urography	Renal computed tomography (CT) scan
	Peritoneal lavage

These tests can reveal rib fractures, delayed or nonvisualized kidney, extravasation of contrast media, renal vessel damage, hematoma, lacerations, infarcts, or free blood in peritoneum.

MEDICAL MANAGEMENT

The goal of care is to maintain renal tissue perfusion and preserve renal tissue.

General management: Depends on the extent of the injury. Minor injuries care similar to that after a renal biopsy (see page 35). Conservative management includes close observation of the patient who is kept on bed rest. Bleeding stops spontaneously.

Surgery: Major/critical renal trauma is an acute emergency requiring immediate diagnosis and intervention because of the possibility of severe, hidden blood loss and acute renal failure. Surgical exploration of the abdomen is indicated with penetrating injuries. The transabdominal approach permits examination of other abdominal organs. Both liver and spleen often are injured, too. Major damage to the kidney may require total or partial nephrectomy (see page 165).

Adjunctive therapy: If acute renal failure develops, hemodialysis may be indicated (see page 134).

Nursing management: Assess for hemodynamic compromise, minimize hazards of diagnostic testing, limit potential for infection. Watch for gradual loss of renal function.

COMPLICATIONS

Subcapsular hematoma	Hemorrhage and shock
Extravasation of urine into perirenal space	Kidney destruction
Retroperitoneal and perinephric hematomas (may be large)	Sepsis, abscess
	Loss of renal function

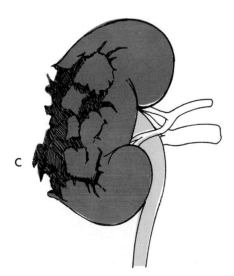

C

Fragmentation

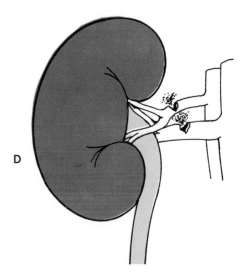

D

Major vascular injury

Extracorporeal Shock-Wave Lithotripsy

Extracorporeal shock-wave lithotripsy (ESWL) is a noninvasive method of treating renal calculi. Carefully directed shock waves enter the body through a liquid medium surrounding the body and disintegrate the calculus; the pulverized material is flushed by the normal excretion of urine.

Fluoroscopy or ultrasonography are used to pinpoint the stone's location. Radiopaque stones are seen easily; radiolucent stones are visualized by using a contrast medium in the renal pelvis. The patient is given general anesthesia and then positioned in the lithotriptor tub, which is filled with treated (degassed, deionized) water (Figures 11-14 and 11-15). After a series of 200 shock waves has been delivered, fluoroscopy is used to determine the location and size of the stone fragments or gravel. The number of shocks needed depends on the size of the stone; an average treatment is 1,000 to 2,000 shocks, with a maximum of 2,400 per treatment. If the gravel formed blocks the ureter, a percutaneous nephrostomy may be done to promote clearance of the particles.

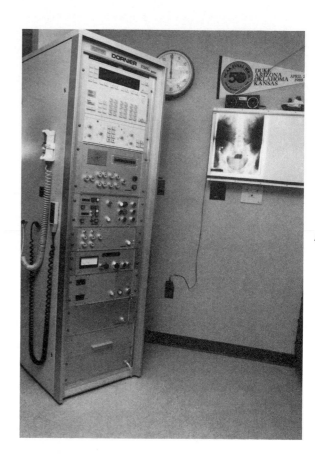

A

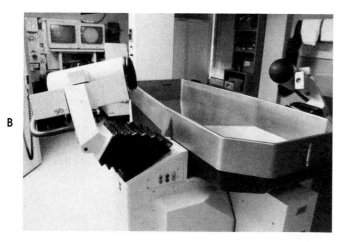

B

FIGURE 11-14.
A, ESWL control panel and x-ray (see stones in left kidney and marker on right). **B,** Tub for extracorporeal shock-wave lithotripsy (ESWL). **C,** Source of impulse located in bottom of tub.

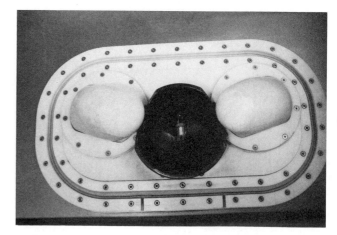

C

PROCEDURAL GUIDELINES

1. Explain the procedure to the patient and family.
2. Prepare the patient for general anesthesia.
3. Any urinary tract infection is treated and antibiotics are given before the procedure if an infected stone is to be pulverized.

INDICATIONS

Stones of appropriate size, type, and location
Noninvasive treatment desirable
No correctable anatomic abnormalities

CONTRAINDICATIONS AND CAUTIONS

Pregnancy
Lower ureteral stones
Bladder stones
Cardiac pacemakers
Distal ureteral obstruction
Renal artery calcifications
Bleeding diatheses

COMPLICATIONS

Hematuria
Ureteral colic
Ureteral obstruction

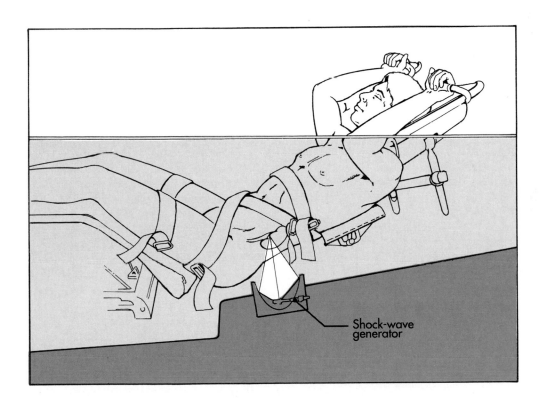

FIGURE 11 15
Patient positioned for shock-wave lithotripsy. Area of flank is exposed for efficient shock-wave conduction.

1 ASSESS

ASSESSMENT	OBSERVATIONS
Urinary tract	Hematuria for 12-24 hr; passage of stone particles
General	Pain of passage of stone fragments (ureteral colic); fever, increased WBC, pyuria, bacteriuria

2 DIAGNOSE

NURSING DIAGNOSIS	SUPPORTIVE ASSESSMENT FINDINGS
Altered patterns of urinary elimination related to passage of stone particles	Hematuria, stone particles in urine
Pain related to passage of stone particles	Patient complains of pain in flank, extending to groin and labia or testicle; guarding behavior noted
Potential for infection related to infected stone	Fever, leukocytosis, pyuria, bacteriuria, dysuria

3 PLAN

Patient goals

1. The patient will have normal urinary elimination patterns.
2. The patient will be free of pain.
3. The patient will be free of infection.
4. The patient will be knowledgeable about renal calculi and will understand home care and necessary follow-up medical care.

4 IMPLEMENT

NURSING DIAGNOSIS	NURSING INTERVENTIONS	RATIONALE
Altered patterns of urinary elimination related to passage of stone particles	Assess intake and output and nature of urine.	To identify urinary tract obstruction and monitor the amount of hematuria.
	Strain all urine.	To observe the nature and size of particles being passed.
	Ensure adequate fluid intake.	Extra fluids may be needed to help the passage of stone particles.
Pain related to passage of stone particles	Assess for pain; give analgesic drugs as ordered; monitor and record response. Use nonpharmacologic methods such as external application of heat.	To determine need for drug, provide relief, and monitor response, including side effects.

NURSING DIAGNOSIS	NURSING INTERVENTIONS	RATIONALE
	Help patient walk, if appropriate.	To help stones move by gravity.
Potential for infection related to infected stone	Assess temperature q 4 hr; monitor WBC and urinalysis for pyuria and bacteriuria.	To identify any infection promptly.
Knowledge deficit	See Patient Teaching.	

5 EVALUATE

PATIENT OUTCOME	DATA INDICATING THAT OUTCOME IS REACHED
Urinary pattern has returned to normal.	Patient has no signs or symptoms of urinary tract infection or obstruction.
Patient is free of pain.	Patient does not complain of pain.
Patient is free of infection.	No signs or symptoms of infection are noted.
Patient and family are knowledgeable about renal calculi and ESWL.	Patient and family understand renal calculi, home care, and follow-up medical care.

PATIENT TEACHING

1. Explain the procedure for extracorporeal shock-wave lithotripsy.
2. Explain the necessary preparation for general anesthesia.
3. Explain the postprocedure care and the possibility of hematuria for 12 to 24 hours, the passage of stone particles, the need to strain urine, and the need to drink extra fluids.
4. Explain how to prevent recurrence of the particular type of stone involved. (See "Renal Calculi," page 99, and Patient Teaching Guide, "Preventing Recurrence of Kidney Stones," page 181).

CHAPTER 12

Patient Teaching Guides

Nurses play an important role in patient education. With more complex diagnostic and treatment programs, patients often face the need to learn about strange equipment and unfamiliar procedures. Compounding these problems is the shortened hospital stay for most patients.

Written materials can help patients understand their treatments and what they must do to manage at home. Specific materials that explain life on dialysis or after transplantation are used by nurses who care for these special patients. Frequently, more general explanations are needed for patients early in the course of renal or urinary system disease. Materials included here give an overview of areas of interest for such patients. These instructions may be copied and given to patients and families.

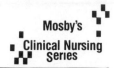
Preventing Urinary Tract Infections

Urinary tract infection (UTI) is a broad term describing any infection or inflammation located along the urinary tract. Most urinary tract infections develop in the bladder or urethra, the canal that carries the urine from the bladder to the urethral opening.

What causes urinary tract infections?

Urinary tract infections result from a number of causes. Most such infections are caused by bacteria from the bowel that have invaded the urinary tract. Because a woman's urethra is closer to the rectum than a man's is, women suffer many more urinary tract infections. Other causes include overstretching of the bladder, urine left in the bladder (incomplete voiding), and lack of cleanliness during catheterization. Urethral inflammation can be caused by chemical irritants such as perfumed feminine hygiene products, sanitary napkins, spermicidal foams and jellies, and bubble bath.

What are the signs of a urinary tract infection?

Several signs indicate a urinary tract infection. You may have just one symptom or a combination of the following:
1. Frequent and urgent need to urinate
2. Pain in the lower back and lower pelvic region
3. Cloudy or foul-smelling urine
4. Bloody urine
5. Chills or fever
6. Lack of appetite and/or lack of energy

How to prevent a urinary tract infection or inflammation

The two most important things you can do to prevent a urinary tract infection are to practice good hygiene and drink plenty of fluids. Women should avoid wiping fecal matter into the urethral area. Wiping from front to back will help prevent germs and bacteria from entering the urethral opening. Showering or bathing daily also helps prevent the spread of germs into the urinary tract.

Drinking lots of fluids helps the bladder rid itself of bacteria. However, certain liquids may irritate the bladder, such as carbonated beverages, coffee, tea, and alcoholic drinks.

Urinate on a regular basis during waking hours, every 2 to 3 hours to avoid overstretching the bladder. Never postpone urination for a period of 8 hours or longer to finish your work shift.

To prevent inflammation of the urethral opening, avoid perfumed feminine hygiene products and bubble bath. Wash the perineal area after using spermicidal jelly or foam.

See your health professional if you think you might have a urinary tract infection. Such infections can lead to bladder and kidney damage, kidney stones, and urine retention.

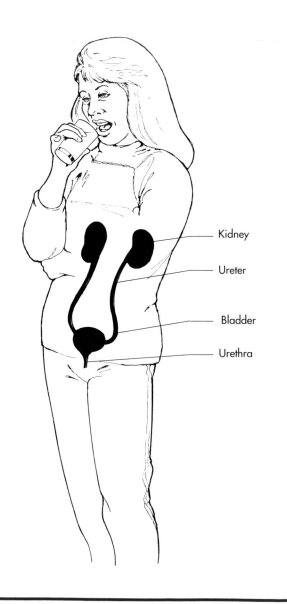

Kidney

Ureter

Bladder

Urethra

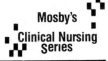
Preventing Recurrence of Kidney Stones

Passing a kidney stone can be a very painful experience. Anyone who has experienced the agony of passing a stone is eager never to endure such pain again. Fortunately, some measures can help prevent the recurrence of kidney stones.

What are kidney stones?

Just as the name implies, kidney stones are small, gravelly stones formed in the kidney. Kidney stones are usually made up of uric acid or calcium but sometimes may contain oxalate. After the stone matures in the kidney, it passes down the ureter into the bladder and then out the urethra. It is this movement that causes the pain. Sometimes the stone is too large to be passed through the urinary tract and must be removed surgically.

What causes kidney stones?

A number of factors can cause kidney stones. These include:

- *Heredity.* If someone in your immediate family has had kidney stones, you have an increased chance of also having kidney stones.
- *Injury.* Sometimes an injury to the kidney can cause a stone to form.
- *Biochemical imbalances.* Some people have too much calcium in their bodies, and some of this calcium forms stones.
- *Diseases.* Diseases such as hyperparathyroidism, hyperthyroidism, and certain types of cancer can cause kidney stones. Patients with gout have too much uric acid in their blood and have a greater chance of forming uric acid kidney stones.
- *Gender and age.* Men have a greater chance of forming kidney stones than do women. Most men who get kidney stones are between 20 and 50 years of age.
- *Diet.* People who eat foods high in oxalate (such as okra) and calcium seem to have an increased risk of developing kidney stones. Too much salt may also be a factor.
- *Urine.* Some people's urine is very concentrated or alkaline; this can lead to kidney stone formation.

- *Not drinking enough water.* When you don't drink enough water, your urine becomes very concentrated, which can lead to the formation of stones. People who live in an area with very hot summers or who have jobs in which they perspire a lot have an increased risk of developing stones.
- *Urinary tract infections.* People who have urinary tract infections are more likely to have kidney stones.
- *Medications.* Certain medications can cause kidney stones to form. Too much vitamin C has been found to enhance stone formation.
- *Postpregnancy.* Many women get kidney stones after giving birth. The reason has not been discovered yet, although some doctors suspect hormonal changes or the addition of calcium to the diet.

Sometimes it is a combination of these factors that is causing your kidney stones.

How do we prevent kidney stones from recurring?

The best treatment for kidney stones is to prevent them from recurring. If possible, your doctor will try to determine what kind of kidney stone you had. He or she will then explain to you how to best prevent any more stones from developing. Some of the preventions may include:

- *Drinking lots of fluids, especially water.* Keep your body well hydrated to prevent concentrated urine and stone formation. Drinking cranberry juice can help people whose urine is too alkaline.
- *Avoiding foods high in oxalate.* If your stones are formed of oxalates, you may need to cut out certain foods from your diet, such as tea, chocolate, nuts, and spinach.
- *Avoiding foods high in uric acid.* If your stones are caused by excess uric acid, you will need to reduce the foods you eat that are high in uric acid such as organ meats, shrimp, and dried beans.
- *Restricting milk and milk products.* If your stones are formed from calcium, you may need to cut back on your calcium intake. Cutting back on milk and other products high in calcium may help prevent calcium stones.
- *Changing medication.* If a medication seems to be causing stones to form, your doctor may change your medication.

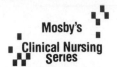

High Blood Pressure and Kidney Disease

Nearly 35 million Americans have high blood pressure (hypertension). High blood pressure is a major cause of heart attacks and stroke. But high blood pressure, left untreated, can also cause kidney disease by narrowing the blood vessels in the kidneys. The kidneys become increasingly unable to process fluids and waste products from the blood. Eventually the kidneys fail.

What is high blood pressure?

When a nurse or doctor takes your blood pressure, he or she is measuring the force of your blood on the walls of your artery right after your heart beats (systolic blood pressure) and in between heart beats (diastolic blood pressure). The systolic pressure number is the highest and the diastolic pressure number is the lowest. A blood pressure of less than 140/90 is considered normal blood pressure. A blood pressure of between 140/90 and 160/95 is considered borderline high blood pressure. Any blood pressure reading over 160/95 is considered high blood pressure.

What causes high blood pressure?

The cause of high blood pressure is unknown, but certain risk factors can lead to high blood pressure in some people. The following is a list of these risk factors:

- A family history of high blood pressure
- Age—people over 50 years of age have a greater chance of developing high blood pressure, although it can occur at any age
- Race—blacks have a higher incidence of high blood pressure and a greater risk for developing kidney disease as a result
- Obesity
- Stress
- Cigarette smoking
- A diet high in salt and saturated fats

How is high blood pressure treated?

Some risk factors, such as family history, race, and age, cannot be changed. However, other risk factors can be controlled. Almost all patients are told to cut back on salt and satu-rated fats. Patients who are overweight are put on calorie-controlled diets so they can lose excess weight. Patients who smoke are advised to stop or at least to cut back on the number of cigarettes they smoke. If stress appears to be the reason for the high blood pressure reading, patients are taught relaxation techniques, and they are advised to try to avoid the things causing them stress (although this isn't always possible.) Exercise is also an important part of keeping blood pressure down.

Sometimes, however, these methods are not enough to lower blood pressure; then medication becomes necessary. There are many types of high blood pressure medication available, and your doctor will prescribe the one that will best treat your high blood pressure. It is extremely important that you take your medication every day, no matter how you feel. High blood pressure sometimes has no symptoms. You may feel fine but still have high blood pressure.

What else should I know about high blood pressure and kidney disease?

Some people who already have kidney disease develop high blood pressure. Almost all people whose kidneys have completely failed and who undergo dialysis have high blood pressure. The treatment for high blood pressure caused by kidney disease is very similar to the treatment described above. However, people with kidney disease must also restrict the amount of protein and potassium in their diets and restrict their fluid intake.

Outlook

Often high blood pressure is discovered during routine physical examinations. If you are diagnosed with high blood pressure, it is important that you follow your doctor's instructions about diet and medication to prevent possible kidney disease. It is also important that you see your doctor regularly, because your high blood pressure must be closely monitored.

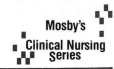
Diabetes and Kidney Disease

A patient who has diabetes runs a greater risk of developing kidney disease, especially if the diabetes started before the patient was 20 years old (juvenile-onset diabetes). Diabetes can cause vascular changes that can affect the kidneys' function; they become less and less able to process and metabolize carbohydrates, proteins, fats, and insulin. The level of kidney function usually decreases gradually until the kidneys stop functioning altogether.

To help prevent the loss of kidney function, it is important that you prevent high blood pressure and maintain good control of your blood sugar level. The more your blood sugar level fluctuates, the harder your kidneys have to work. Keep your blood sugar at the level that your doctor prescribes, and you will help slow kidney deterioration.

What happens if you do develop kidney disease?

Even with careful monitoring and proper preventive measures, many people with diabetes develop kidney disease. If this happens, your doctor may instruct you to either increase or decrease the amount of insulin you take each day. You also may need to take antihypertensive drugs to control high blood pressure and diuretics to help eliminate excess fluids from your body. Your doctor may prescribe other drugs as well.

For the most part you can continue to follow your normal diabetic diet, with only a few changes. Your doctor may instruct you to restrict the amount of protein, sodium, and potassium in your diet. Your fluid intake may also be restricted. These restrictions are necessary, because your kidneys cannot process protein, sodium, potassium, and fluids as well as they used to. However, you must be sure to get the right amount of calories. A dietitian will develop a meal plan for you that will take care of your nutritional needs.

Because the kidneys aren't functioning properly, infection becomes a serious concern. You may become susceptible to viral, bacterial, and fungal infections. These infections can be serious, and you must learn to recognize their signs and symptoms:

- Fever over 100° F
- Redness, swelling, or pain around any wound
- Coughing, sore throat, and stuffy or runny nose
- Nausea, vomiting, or diarrhea
- Chest pain or shortness of breath
- Burning or frequency of urination or a change in the color or odor of the urine
- Sores or white patches in the mouth

Call your doctor immediately if you have any of these signs or symptoms.

Personal hygiene can go a long way toward preventing infection. Here are some health habits you should follow:

- Take a bath or shower every day.
- Use lotion to lubricate dry skin.
- Don't scratch bites or rashes, since this may lead to infection.
- Use topical antibiotics on minor skin wounds.
- Avoid people with colds.
- Wash your hands.
- Tell your dentist that you have diabetes and kidney failure. You may need to take antibiotics before undergoing any dental work.

You need to balance rest with exercise. Walking is good, easy exercise that can help your blood circulation.

Some patients with diabetes eventually experience total kidney failure. These patients have to begin some form of dialysis, either hemodialysis or peritoneal dialysis. A kidney and pancreas transplant, which can restore kidney function and insulin production, may become an alternative for these patients.

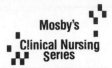

Polycystic Kidney Disease

Polycystic kidney disease is an inherited condition in which the kidney tissue is replaced by grapelike clusters of cysts. Why these cysts occur is unclear, but as they grow larger, they compress and destroy the healthy kidney tissue. As the disease progresses, kidney stones may form, and the kidneys become susceptible to infection. Antibiotics have trouble fighting these infections, because pockets of bacteria form around the cysts. High blood pressure occurs, because the kidneys aren't working right. Kidney failure usually occurs within 5 to 15 years after the first symptoms appear.

Who gets polycystic kidney disease?

The patient with polycystic kidney disease has inherited the dominant gene for the disease from one of his or her parents. The symptoms usually do not become apparent until the patient is 40 years old or older, but they can occur any time between the ages of 20 and 80. The disease affects both men and women.

What are the symptoms of polycystic kidney disease?

The signs and symptoms of polycystic kidney disease are:

- A dull or acute pain in the lower back over the kidney area
- Blood in the urine
- Frequent infections
- High blood pressure
- Enlarged kidneys
- Decreased kidney function

What are the medical treatments for polycystic kidney disease?

No medical treatment can prevent or halt polycystic kidney disease. Draining the cysts doesn't prevent them from growing back and sometimes leads to infection. The best management of this disease includes preventing high blood pressure and infection; this helps preserve kidney function as long as possible.

High blood pressure can best be prevented by cutting back on salt intake and keeping your weight down. Avoiding stress and taking time to relax can also help keep blood pressure from ris-

ing. Sometimes, however, these measures aren't enough. Your doctor may have to prescribe medication to help lower your blood pressure.

Patients with polycystic kidney disease run a greater risk of developing urinary tract infections, and you need to be able to recognize the signs of such an infection. You may have one or a combination of symptoms:

- Frequent and urgent need to urinate
- Pain in the lower back and lower pelvic region
- Cloudy or foul-smelling urine
- Bloody urine
- Chills or fever
- Lack of appetite or lack of energy, or both

The most important thing you can do to prevent a urinary tract infection is to practice good hygiene. Women should avoid wiping fecal matter into the urethral area. Wiping from front to back will help prevent germs and bacteria from entering the urethral opening. Showering or bathing daily also will help prevent the spread of germs.

Drinking lots of fluids helps the bladder flush itself. Urinating when you first feel the urge will help prevent overstretching of the bladder.

Even if you have no symptoms of polycystic kidney disease yet, you will need to have a creatinine clearance test and urine cultures done every 6 months. If symptoms appear, you must be monitored more closely and have tests done more often.

When the disease has progressed to the point of total kidney failure, you will have to begin some form of dialysis, either hemodialysis or peritoneal dialysis. A kidney transplant, which can restore kidney function, may become an alternative.

Genetic counseling is advised for those who have a family history of polycystic kidney disease.

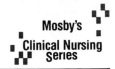
Chronic Renal Disease

Your kidneys perform crucial functions that affect all parts of your body. Your kidneys, in fact, keep the rest of your body in balance and working properly. When chronic renal (kidney) disease causes the kidneys to fail, your whole body stops functioning correctly, and you can become extremely ill unless the condition is treated.

How do the kidneys function?

The kidneys are located at the bottom of the rib cage, one on each side of the spine. Each is about the size of a fist and contains about a million functioning units, called **nephrons.** The nephrons' job is to cleanse the blood of toxic wastes and excess fluid and to add needed chemicals such as hormones and vitamins. The cleansed blood is then returned to the bloodstream. About 200 quarts of fluid are filtered through the kidneys every 24 hours. Of this fluid, 2 quarts are eliminated as urine and the rest is retained in the body.

The kidneys are responsible for regulating the body's salt, potassium, and acid content. They also control the production of red blood cells and regulate blood pressure.

What causes chronic renal disease?

There are several different types and causes of chronic renal disease. **Glomerulonephritis,** which can arise from a number of immune disorders, is an inflammation of the kidney and can damage the nephrons. **High blood pressure,** whether a result of kidney disorder or a cause of kidney disease, can hasten kidney failure. **Diabetes mellitus** may cause kidney disease. **Polycystic kidney disease** is an inherited disorder in which cysts form on kidney tissue and eventually destroy the healthy kidney tissue. **Congenital anomalies** can cause obstructions, which can lead to infection and destruction of kidney tissue. **Interstitial nephritis,** usually caused by drug use, is an inflammation of kidney tissue and leads to eventual destruction of the kidney. **Nephrotic syndrome** can occur with a variety of kidney problems, including glomerulonephritis, diabetes, and infections.

What are the signs of renal failure?

Because kidney failure sometimes gives no warning signs, it can go undiagnosed until it is well advanced. However, there are six warning signs of kidney disease that you should be aware of:
1. High blood pressure
2. Puffiness around the eyes and swelling in the hands and feet (edema)
3. Pain in the kidney area (the small of the back just below the ribs)
4. Difficulty urinating or burning during urination
5. More frequent urination and urinating during the night
6. Passage of bloody or cola-colored urine

How is renal failure treated?

When kidney failure is in its early stage, it may be slowed by special diets or medication or both. However, as the disease progresses and the kidneys no longer perform their duties of removing bodily wastes, other treatments must be used. The blood must be cleansed by using an artificial kidney *(hemodialysis)* or by introducing a cleansing solution into the abdomen *(peritoneal dialysis).* A *kidney transplant,* in which a healthy, donated kidney replaces the failed kidneys, can restore normal kidney function.

Outlook

There is no cure for chronic renal disease. Following the program your doctor prescribes for you is vitally important to helping you live with kidney failure. Thousands of people who have the disease are living active, productive lives.

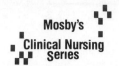

Renal Diet

Diet is very important for patients with renal (kidney) disorders. Because the kidneys cannot get rid of enough fluids and waste products, certain foods and liquids must be controlled. Controlling the amount of protein, calories, potassium, sodium, and fluids that you take in every day can help lessen your kidneys' workload, can make you feel less nauseated, and can boost your energy level.

Protein

Protein is important for building muscles and repairing tissues. People with kidney disorders, however, usually need to limit the amount of protein they consume, because the kidneys cannot rid the body of excess protein waste products.

There are two types of protein, *high-quality protein* and *low-quality protein.*

1. High-quality protein comes from animals and includes meat, chicken, fish, and eggs. You should eat high-quality protein at every meal.

2. Low-quality protein comes from plants and includes grains and vegetables. You need to limit how much low-quality protein you eat.

Calories

You need to consume enough calories every day to maintain your energy and prevent weight loss. Most of your calories should come from carbohydrates and unsaturated fats. If you need to increase your caloric intake, try adding margarine and oils that are low in cholesterol and jams, jellies, sugar, and honey to your diet.

Potassium

It is very important to control the amount of potassium in your diet. Too little potassium can cause muscle weakness, fatigue, and irregular heartbeats. Too much potassium can cause heart problems and even death.

Certain foods contain large amounts of potassium. These include dried beans, nuts, meat, fruits, vegetables, and milk. Salt substitutes also contain a large amount of potassium.

Sodium

Sodium can be found in a number of foods. Table salt and some prepared and packaged foods are very high in sodium.

Too much sodium will cause your body to retain fluid. Try using herbs and spices instead of salt to season your food.

Fluid

Fluid is anything you drink, of course, but it also includes things such as ice, gelatin, and ice cream—anything that is liquid at room temperature.

Too much fluid can cause a number of problems, including weight gain, swelling (edema), high blood pressure, shortness of breath, fluid in the lungs, and heart failure.

The amount of fluid you're allowed will depend on how much kidney function you have left.

Vitamins and minerals

The amount you get of some vitamins and minerals may also need to be controlled. These nutrients may include folic acid; vitamins A, B, C, and D; calcium; iron; zinc; aluminum; and phosphorus.

The renal diet your physician prescribes for you will depend on how much kidney function you have left. If you need to undergo peritoneal dialysis or hemodialysis, or if you have a kidney transplant, your diet will need to be adjusted.

Your dietitian will help you plan your diet. She can tell you where to buy special foods and how to read the labels on prepared foods. Follow your physician's instructions and your diet, and you will be doing the best thing for your body and helping yourself feel better.

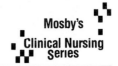

Mosby's
**Clinical Nursing
Series**

What is Hemodialysis?

Hemodialysis is just one of the possible treatments for patients whose kidneys have stopped working, either temporarily or permanently. Hemodialysis involves cleansing the patient's blood of harmful toxins and excess fluid in an artificial kidney machine and returning the clean blood to the patient.

Before beginning dialysis, an **access** must be prepared in your arm or leg. A surgeon will create an internal **fistula** in your arm or leg to allow access for the removal and return of blood during the hemodialysis treatment. A fistula is formed by joining a vein and an artery to make an enlarged vessel. After the fistula heals, two needles are placed in the vessel, one on the artery side and one on the vein side. The needles are attached to plastic tubing that leads into the artificial kidney. Dialysis can now begin.

How does an artificial kidney (hemodialyzer) work?

The machine that cleans the blood is called a **hemodialyzer.** It acts as an artificial kidney. The hemodialyzer has two compartments that are separated by a thin, porous (semipermeable) membrane. One compartment is for blood; the other is for a solution called dialysate. As your blood is pumped through the machine, the dialysate solution is also pumped into the machine, where wastes move from your blood to the dialysate. The dialysate solution is specially formulated to treat each patient's blood and may contain such substances as glucose, potassium, or sodium acetate. The smaller waste products in the blood and the excess fluids are passed through the semipermeable membrane and washed away.

If you experience nausea, vomiting, dizziness, faintness, or headache during hemodialysis, notify your doctor or nurse. You may be experiencing overly rapid fluid loss. It is normal to feel tired after a hemodialysis treatment. You should feel better the next day.

How long does hemodialysis treatment last, and how often is it necessary?

The treatment process takes about 3 to 4 hours, depending on how much kidney function you have left and how much excess fluid and toxins have built up in your blood. Hemodialysis is usually done three times a week.

Where does hemodialysis take place?

Hemodialysis can be done in the hospital, a free-standing dialysis unit, or at home. There are advantages and disadvantages to each location. A hospital or dialysis unit has trained personnel to do your treatment, but you have to adhere to the unit or hospital's schedule. Just getting there may be a problem. Home dialysis offers you the convenience of having your own machine and doing the procedure yourself (with the help of a partner) at a time that is convenient for you. However, sometimes home dialysis can add to family stress. Your doctor and you can decide together where your hemodialysis should take place.

Diet and medication

You will probably have restrictions on the amount of salt (sodium), potassium, and protein you can have. Too much or too little of these substances can cause problems for a dialysis patient, some of them serious. It is important that you follow the diet guidelines your doctor gives you.

Many dialysis patients also have restrictions on their fluid intake. Fluids can build up between dialysis treatments and can cause high blood pressure and swelling, along with more serious complications. It is very important that you follow your doctor's guidelines as to your fluid intake.

Medication may be prescribed for you. It is important that you know when to take your medicine, and how much you should take. Don't take any medication, including over-the-counter medicines, that your doctor has not prescribed.

Outlook

Hemodialysis takes over the kidneys' function but does not cure kidney failure. If your kidney failure is chronic, you will have to undergo some form of dialysis for the rest of your life or until you receive a kidney transplant. Many patients lead near-normal lives despite hemodialysis except for the need to have the treatments.

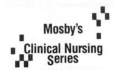

What Is Peritoneal Dialysis?

Peritoneal dialysis is one method of removing waste products and excess fluids from the blood when the kidneys stop functioning. Unlike hemodialysis, which is done with an artificial kidney machine, peritoneal dialysis is carried out in the patient's own body.

How does peritoneal dialysis work?

Peritoneal dialysis takes place in your abdomen. A membrane, called the peritoneal membrane, surrounds your intestines and acts as a filtering membrane. A dialysate solution flows into the abdomen, where harmful toxins and excess fluids move from the blood to the dialysate. The solution is then drained out of the abdomen.

Before peritoneal dialysis can begin, a tube (catheter) will be inserted into the peritoneal cavity in your abdomen through a small incision. When the catheter is in place, you will have three types of peritoneal dialysis from which to choose: *continuous ambulatory peritoneal dialysis, continuous cycling peritoneal dialysis,* and *intermittent peritoneal dialysis.*

Continuous ambulatory peritoneal dialysis (CAPD) is done without the use of any machines. A bag of dialysate solution is warmed to body temperature. Then, while you sit or lie down, the solution flows into your abdomen through tubing that connects the catheter in your abdomen to the bag of dialysate. This takes about 10 minutes. The bag is hung on a stand so it is at a higher level than your abdomen.

After the solution is drained into your abdomen, you clamp the tubing, roll up the empty bag and tuck it into your clothing. Then you go about your normal daily activities. Four to 8 hours later, the dialysate solution must be drained out of your abdomen back into the bag. Again, sit or lie down while this occurs, but this time the bag must be lower than your abdomen. It takes about 10 to 20 minutes to drain out. A new bag of dialysate then flows into your abdomen, and the process begins anew. This process usually is repeated three to four times during the day and once at night.

Continuous cycling peritoneal dialysis (CCPD) takes place while you sleep, using a cycling machine. Before you go to sleep, you hook tubing from the machine to the catheter in your abdomen. Three to seven times during the night, the continuous cycling machine automatically drains dialysate solution into your abdomen and back out again. During the last run, the solution is left in your abdomen and will remain there during the day. It will be drained the following night. When you wake the next morning, you disconnect the tubing and go about your daily activities.

Intermittent peritoneal dialysis (IPD) is usually done in the hospital, three to five times a week. You will be dialyzed by a machine that takes 8 to 12 hours to complete a treatment. Treatment is usually carried out while you sleep.

Complications

Patients undergoing peritoneal dialysis are at some risk of developing an infection of the abdomen called *peritonitis.* If you experience abdominal pain or fever or notice that the dialysate solution that drains back into the bag or machine is cloudy, notify your doctor at once. Diarrhea, vomiting, and a swollen abdomen can also be signs of peritonitis and should be reported to your doctor.

Outlook

Peritoneal dialysis takes over the kidneys' function but does not cure kidney failure. You will need to undergo some form of dialysis for the rest of your life or until you receive a kidney transplant. Many patients lead near normal lives despite peritoneal dialysis except for the need to have the treatments and some restrictions on food and fluid intake.

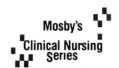
Preparing for a Kidney Transplant

A renal (kidney) transplant is the surgical placement of a donor kidney into a patient whose kidneys no longer work. The donor kidney takes over all the functions that the patient's diseased and damaged kidneys used to perform when they were healthy. These functions include producing urine, removing waste products and excess fluid, and regulating blood pressure, red blood cell production, and the fluids and chemicals the body needs.

Your donor kidney may come from a living relative or from a recently deceased person (cadaver). In either case, the donated kidney must be compatible so that your body doesn't reject it immediately. Your doctor will perform tests on both you and the donor to make sure your tissues and blood types match.

Transplant surgery—what to expect

It is best to undergo hemodialysis the day before surgery to ensure that your body fluids and electrolytes are in balance. However, if your donated kidney is coming from a cadaver, you may not have time. Kidneys must be transplanted within 24 to 72 hours of removal, or they are useless.

If there is time, you will be given drugs to help lessen the possibility of your body's rejecting the new kidney.

Before surgery can begin, a few procedures must be done, including blood tests, electrocardiograms (heart monitoring), chest x-rays, and a complete physical examination. You will not be allowed to eat or drink anything for several hours before your surgery. Again, if your kidney comes from a cadaver, you may not have very much notice before surgery and may come into the hospital with a full stomach. Your doctor can take precautions if you do.

Shortly before surgery, you will be given medication to make you drowsy and relaxed. After you are taken to the operating room, the anesthesiologist will give you a medication that will make you sleep. Catheters will be placed in your bladder to measure urine output.

An incision about 7 inches long will be made, and the donated kidney will be implanted. The operation takes about 3 to 4 hours. Your diseased kidneys probably will not be removed. Sometimes the nonfunctioning kidneys must be removed (e.g., if they are infected).

After surgery

You will be in a special care unit for a few days after surgery. Catheters will remain in your bladder and kidney for 7 days or so to monitor how much urine your new kidney is producing. Don't be alarmed if your urine is pink tinged or bloody at first; this is normal. Your nurses will be monitoring your condition very carefully.

Your new kidney should start functioning immediately. Sometimes, however, the donor kidney goes into a kind of shock and needs some time to "wake up." This waking-up period may take anywhere from a few days to a few months. Until the new kidney starts working, you will have to continue undergoing kidney dialysis.

Rejection

Your body considers your new kidney a foreign body and will try to reject it. For this reason your doctor will prescribe drugs to suppress your immune system. You will have to take these drugs for the rest of your life. If you stop taking them, your body will reject your new kidney.

Even if you take your drugs properly, you may experience a rejection episode. The chances of rejection are highest in the first few months after transplantation, although there is always the possibility of rejection. The signs of kidney rejection are:
- Soreness or pain in the kidney area
- Fever over 100° F
- Decrease in urine output
- Sudden weight gain or swelling or both
- Increased blood pressure
- Flulike symptoms, including nausea, vomiting, and diarrhea

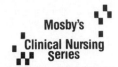
Going Home After a Kidney Transplant

You will be allowed to go home 2 to 3 weeks after surgery. You should avoid any heavy lifting for the next 2 to 3 months. Avoid contact sports, but do make walking part of your daily routine. You should be able to return to your job about 6 weeks after surgery.

Although the drugs you will be taking can cause some undesirable side effects, your new kidney can return your life to near normal. Dialysis will no longer be needed, and you should have fewer dietary and fluid restrictions. Also, you will feel better and have more energy.

Your renal (kidney) transplantation is over, and you've been discharged from the hospital. Your home care is now beginning, and there are some things you need to know about taking care of yourself and monitoring your new kidney's function.

Keeping records

For the first 3 weeks after discharge, you will need to keep daily records on the following:

1. *Daily urine output.* You need to measure and record how much urine you produce.

2. *Daily fluid intake.* Measure and record all fluids, including ice.

3. *Weight.* Weigh yourself every morning before eating and after urinating.

4. *Temperature.* Take your temperature at the same time every afternoon. If you begin running a temperature higher than 100° F, call your doctor.

5. *Blood pressure.* Take blood pressure readings every day at the same time and record the readings.

Diet and medication

You should have fewer diet restrictions now than when you were undergoing dialysis, but the immunosuppressive medication you will be taking to prevent kidney rejection can cause some side effects that can be controlled by diet. *Cyclosporine* can raise potassium levels, and you may have to restrict your potassium intake. *Prednisone* can cause salt retention, increased appetite, and an increase in your blood sugar level.

You may need to follow a low-sodium, low-calorie, and/or restricted-sugar diet.

Cyclosporine and prednisone have other side effects. Cyclosporine can cause flushing, hair growth on the face and body, gum swelling, headaches, high blood pressure, and kidney toxicity. Prednisone can cause rounding of the face and abdomen, increased sweating, easy bruising, acne, muscle weakness, cataracts, joint pain, delayed wound healing, and restlessness or moodiness.

Another immunosuppressive drug is *azathioprine.* Azathioprine can decrease your white blood cell count and cause temporary hair loss.

The side effects of these drugs are usually not too troublesome, and some can be controlled. After a few months, when the dosage is lowered, some of these side effects may decrease or disappear.

You must take your immunosuppressive medication for the rest of your life. If you stop, your body will reject your new kidney. Notify your doctor if you forget to take your medication.

If you are taking prednisone, your doctor may also tell you to take an antacid when you take the prednisone to help prevent stomach irritation.

You should never take aspirin, since it can cause stomach bleeding. You may take acetaminophen (Tylenol) for pain. Check with your doctor before you take any prescriptive or over-the-counter drug.

Health habits

Personal hygiene is very important. Here are some health habits you should follow:

- Take a bath or shower every day.
- Use lotion to lubricate dry skin.
- Don't scratch bites or rashes, since this may lead to infection.
- Use topical antibiotics on minor skin wounds.
- Avoid people with colds.
- Wash your hands.
- Tell your dentist that you have had a kidney transplant and are taking immunosuppressive drugs. You may need to take antibiotics before undergoing any dental work.

You must take care of yourself and your new kidney. Avoid any contact sports such as football or hockey but do make walking part of your daily routine. Your doctor may recommend birth control for a period of time.

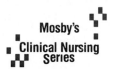

Complications After a Kidney Transplant

Signs of infection

Your doctor has prescribed drugs for you that will help prevent your body from rejecting your new kidney. These drugs work by suppressing your immune system, which has the job of recognizing and destroying things that are foreign to your body (such as your new kidney). However, because the immune system also has the job of fighting off infection, you may become susceptible to viral, bacterial, and fungal infections. These infections can be serious, and you must learn to recognize the signs and symptoms:

- Fever over 100° F
- Redness, swelling, or pain around any wound
- Coughing, sore throat, and stuffy or runny nose
- Nausea, vomiting, or diarrhea
- Chest pain or shortness of breath
- Burning or frequency of urination or a change in the color or odor of the urine
- Sores or white patches in the mouth

Call your doctor immediately if you notice any of these signs or symptoms. After the first few months, your drug dosage should be lowered and the chance of infection will decrease.

Signs of rejection

Your body considers your new kidney a foreign body and will try to reject it. For this reason, the doctor has prescribed drugs that will suppress your immune system. You must take these drugs for the rest of your life. If you stop taking them, your body will reject your new kidney.

Even if you take your drugs properly, you may experience a rejection episode. The chances of rejection are highest in the first few months after transplantation, although there is always the possibility of rejection. The signs of kidney rejection are:

- Soreness or pain in the kidney area
- Fever over 100° F
- Decrease in urine output
- Sudden weight gain or swelling or both
- Increased blood pressure
- Flulike symptoms, including nausea, vomiting, and diarrhea

Notify your doctor immediately if you notice any of these signs or symptoms.

Continuing medical supervision

You will need to make frequent visits to the outpatient clinic, even if you feel fine and are having no problems. It is important that your doctor and nurses monitor how your new kidney is functioning, and how you are responding to your drug therapy. If you are having problems, you will have to see your doctor even more frequently. Once a year or so, you will have a kidney biopsy, in which a tiny piece of your kidney is checked to see how healthy it is.

If you ever have any problems or questions about your health, don't hesitate to call your doctor.

CHAPTER 13

Renal Drugs

SPECIAL CONSIDERATIONS OF PHARMACOTHERAPY IN THE PATIENT WITH CHRONIC RENAL INSUFFICIENCY

With many drugs, the duration and intensity of the pharmacologic actions depend on the amount of renal function the patient still has. This effect is the result of the significant role the kidneys play in the excretion of drugs and their metabolites from the body. The physiologic disturbances resulting from renal insufficiency may also change the effect of medications in other ways, such as altering protein binding or the volume of drug distribution. With drugs excreted entirely by the kidneys, estimation of renal function (as determined by the glomerular filtration rate) can be used to adjust the amount of drug needed to maintain a therapeutic effect without toxicity. Several methods have been suggested for determining appropriate drug dosages in patients with renal insufficiency; however, these formulas may be neither appropriate nor useful, especially in patients whose renal function changes rapidly. The best method

of assuring safe and therapeutic drug levels is to individualize dosage adjustment on the basis of the drug's concentration in the blood. When this is not possible, the dosage or frequency of administration is reduced according to the patient's creatinine clearance. If only the serum creatinine is available, the following formula may be used to estimate creatinine clearance in the patient with steady-state renal function

$$\text{Men:} \quad \frac{\text{Weight (kg)} \times (140 - \text{age})}{72 \times \text{serum creatinine (mg/dl)}}$$
$$\text{Women:} \quad 0.85 \times \text{above value}$$

Table 13-1 lists some common drug groups, dosage adjustments, and dialysis effects used in reduced renal function. In a patient with renal failure, the amount of drug removed through dialysis should be considered when determining dose amount and frequency.

Table 13-1

ALTERATIONS IN DRUG DOSAGE IN REDUCED RENAL FUNCTION

Drug Group	Dialysis effect*	Comments
Aminoglycosides		
Both ototoxic and nephrotoxic After usual loading dose, intervals are increased according to blood levels	Yes (HD, PD)	Absorption of gentamicin is better from intraperitoneal route to blood than vice versa.
Antifungals		
Increase interval	Yes (HD)	Amphotericin B is nephrotoxic.
Antituberculosis drugs		
Increase interval	Yes (HD, PD)	Rifampin may cause acute renal failure.
Cephalosporins		
Usually, increase interval	Yes (HD)	Some cephalosporins may increase serum creatinine.
Penicillins		
Increase interval	Varies (HD)	May or may not need supplement.
Sulfonamides		
Increase interval	Yes (HD)	Sulfamethoxazole, protein binding decreased in uremia. Trimethoprim, may increase serum creatinine.
Other antiinfectives		Avoid methenamine, nalidixic acid, nitrofurantoin.
Analgesics, non-narcotic		
Increase interval	Varies	Hepatic excretion. Acetaminophen metabolites accumulate; nephrotoxic in overdose. Aspirin nephrotoxic in overdose.
Narcotic analgesics		
Decrease dose	No or unknown	Hepatic excretion. May cause excessive sedation and respiratory depression.
Barbiturates		
Decrease dose	Varies	Hepatic excretion. May cause excessive sedation and respiratory depression.
Benzodiazepines		
Decrease dose	No	May cause excess sedation, respiratory depression, and encephalopathy in patients with ESRD. Avoid chloral hydrate, ethchlorvynol (Placidyl), and glutethemide (Doriden). Lithium carbonate is nephrotoxic.
Phenothiazines		
Decrease dose	No	Hepatic excretion. Anticholinergic.
Tricyclic antidepressants		
Decrease dose	No	Hepatic excretion. Anticholinergic.

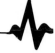

Table 13-1 cont'd

ALTERATIONS IN DRUG DOSAGE IN REDUCED RENAL FUNCTION—cont'd

Drug Group	Dialysis effect*	Comments
Antihypertensives		
Decrease dose or increase interval	Varies	Use blood pressure as guide to dose interval.
Adrenergic modulators: No change or increase interval	Varies	Increase interval for clonidine, methyldopa.
Beta blockers: No change usually	Varies	Atenolol, decrease dose and increase interval.
Angiotensin-converting enzyme inhibitors: Decrease dose	Yes (HD)	Decrease captopril at low GFRs.
Vasodilators: Decrease dose	Yes (HD)	Hydralazine not affected by dialysis.
Antiarrhythmics		
Decrease dose or increase interval	Varies	Blood levels may help to guide therapy. Avoid bretylium.
Cardiac glycosides		
Decrease dose	No	Serum levels best guide to therapy.
Calcium-blocking agents		
Decrease dose	No or unknown	Headaches, dizziness, flushing in renal patients.
Diuretics		
Decrease dose or increase interval.	No or unknown	Avoid acetazolamide, potassium-sparing agents, ethacrynic acid; thiazides ineffective at low GFRs; loop diuretics can augment nephrotoxicity of aminoglycosides. Watch for volume depletion.
Nitrates		
Increase interval	Unknown	Hepatic excretion.
Anticoagulants		
Decrease dose	No or unknown	Titrate carefully to achieve therapeutic effect.
Anticonvulsants		
Decrease dose	Varies	Decreased protein binding in ESRD. Use serum levels to monitor therapy.
Nonsteroidal antiinflammatory agents		
Decrease dose	No	May cause renal dysfunction.
Antineoplastic agents		
Decrease dose and increase interval especially at low GFRs	Varies	Cisplatin, cyclophosphamide, methotrexate, mithracin, streptozocin, vinblastine are nephrotoxic.
Corticosteroids		
Decrease dose	Varies	Watch for azotemia, retention of sodium, glucose intolerance, hypertension.
Hypoglycemic agents		
Decrease dose or increase interval.	No or unknown	Hepatic excretion. Avoid acetohexamide and chlorpropamide.

NOTE: *Yes,* supplement usually needed; *No,* not affected by dialysis; *Varies,* some drugs in category need supplemental dose after dialysis and others do not; *HD,* hemodialysis; *PD,* peritoneal dialysis; *ESRD,* end-stage renal disease; *GFR,* glomerular filtration rate.
Modified from Bennett WM: *Drugs and renal disease,* New York, 1986, Churchill Livingstone.

Table 13-2

LOOP DIURETICS

Generic name	Trade name	Initial dosage	Maximum daily dose	Administration
Bumetanide	Bumex	0.5-2 mg/day	10 mg/day	Oral, IM, IV
Ethacrynic acid	Edecrin	50 mg/day (50 mg IV)	200 mg 2 times/day (100 mg IV)	Oral
Furosemide	Lasix	20-80 mg/day	600 mg/day	Oral, IM, IV

DIURETICS

Drugs that increase renal excretion of water and solutes are called diuretics.

Loop Diuretics

Three diuretic agents are referred to as *loop diuretics*, because they exert their effects primarily on the thick ascending loop of Henle. These agents inhibit reabsorption of sodium and chloride, leading to increased loss of water and potassium. The three loop diuretics, bumetanide (Bumex), ethacrynic acid (Edecrin), and furosemide (Lasix), are the most potent diuretic drugs available. They are structurally different but exert similar effects on the kidneys.

Indications: Edema associated with congestive heart failure (CHF), renal diseases, and other causes. Loop diuretics are the strongest diuretic drugs and are used when potent diuresis is needed or in cases of severe renal insufficiency. Oral forms may be used to treat hypertension, especially when it is associated with CHF, pulmonary edema, or impaired renal function.

Usual dosage: See Table 13-2.

Precautions/contraindications: These drugs should not be used at all or should be used with extreme caution in dehydrated patients or patients in a hepatic coma or severe electrolyte depletion. Hypersensitivity and idiosyncratic reactions, as well as acute allergic interstitial nephritis, have occurred.

Side effects/adverse reactions: Therapy may result in hypovolemia and electrolyte imbalances, including hyponatremia, hypochloremic acidosis, hypokalemia, and hypomagnesemia. Ototoxicity may occur, usually after large doses are administered rapidly intravenously; this may not be reversible. The serum uric acid level may rise during therapy. Furosemide (Lasix) is a sulfonamide derivative, and patients allergic to sulfonamides may show cross-sensitivity.

Pharmacokinetics: A rapid effect is seen after both oral and parenteral administration. The drugs are partially metabolized and primarily excreted through the kidneys.

Interactions: Ototoxicity is increased when these drugs are administered with other ototoxic drugs, such as the aminoglycosides or cisplatin. Potassium loss may increase digitalis toxicity. The effects of lithium are increased by the loop diuretics.

Nursing considerations: Patients' hydration status and electrolyte levels should be monitored. Fluid loss may be monitored by recording fluid intake and output and by periodically weighing the patient. Potassium supplements may be needed to maintain normal potassium levels. Patients receiving digitalis and diuretics are especially prone to digitalis toxicity from hypokalemia and should be closely assessed for signals of digitalis toxicity or hypokalemia. Assess hearing in patients receiving high doses.

Thiazide Diuretics

Hydrochlorothiazide is a prototype of the *thiazide diuretics*. Thiazide diuretics inhibit sodium and chloride reabsorption in the distal tubule. These drugs also decrease calcium excretion. Thiazide diuretics generally exert a sustained, mild effect. The drugs in this class all have a similar maximum effect but vary in dosage and duration of action. They are effective in lowering blood pressure in lower doses, possibly as a result of a vasodilating effect on vascular smooth muscle.

Indications: Thiazide diuretics are primarily used to treat hypertension and congestive heart failure, chronic conditions involving sodium and water retention. Thiazide diuretics are also used to reduce urinary excretion of calcium in patients who form calcium stones.

Usual dosage: See Table 13-3.

Precautions/contraindications: Administer with caution to patients with severe hepatic disease, and monitor closely for potassium or other electrolyte depletion.

Side effects/adverse reactions: Weakness, fatigue, paresthesias, impotence, potassium depletion, and metabolic alkalosis may occur. Reduced glucose tolerance and hyperglycemia may occur, possibly as a result of reduced insulin secretion. The serum uric acid level often

Table 13-3

THIAZIDE DIURETICS

Generic name	Trade names	Initial dosage	Maximum per day	Administration
Benzthiazide (contains tartrazine)	Exna	50-200 mg/day	May be less than initial dose	Oral
Chlorothiazide	Diuril	500 mg-2 g/day in 1 or 2 doses	May be less than initial dose	Oral, IV
Chlorthalidone	Hygroton	25-100 mg/day in one dose	200 mg	Oral
Cyclothiazide	Anhydron	1-2 mg/day	May be less than initial dose	Oral
Hydrochlorothiazide	HydroDiuril Esidrix	25-200 mg in one to three doses	May be less than initial dose	Oral

NOTE: See manufacturers' guidelines for complete dosage information.

rises with thiazide diuretic therapy, which may precipitate gout in some patients.

Pharmacokinetics: Oral preparations are absorbed well and metabolized in varying degrees.

Interactions: Absorption of thiazides is decreased by cholestyramine and colestipol. A synergistic effect is seen when thiazides are administered with loop diuretics or diazoxide. Lithium toxicity is more likely to occur, and hypokalemia may lead to digitalis toxicity.

Nursing considerations: The antihypertensive effects of thiazide diuretics are enhanced if the patient also follows a low-sodium diet. Potassium levels should be monitored, and potassium supplements or high-potassium foods should be added to the diet. A potassium-sparing diuretic may be administered to reduce potassium loss. Glucose levels should be checked in patients with impaired glucose tolerance, and insulin dosage may need to be adjusted for diabetic patients.

Potassium-Sparing Diuretics

Spironolactone (Aldactone) is one of several *potassium-sparing diuretics*. They are competitive antagonists of aldosterone that exert their effects in the collecting tubules. The overall effect is a reduction of potassium and hydrogen ion excretion and a mild increase in sodium excretion. Because of their weak diuretic effects, they are seldom administered alone; rather, they are administered with thiazide diuretics to offset the potassium loss they cause. Because potassium-sparing diuretics have a slow onset of action, several days may pass before the full therapeutic benefit is observed.

Indications: Treatment of hyperaldosteronism and as adjunctive therapy with thiazide or loop diuretics to help prevent diuretic-induced potassium loss.

Usual dosage: See Table 13-4.

Precautions/contraindications: Potassium supplements or a high-potassium diet should *not* be used with potassium-sparing diuretics. The drugs should not be used in cases of chronic renal insufficiency because of increased risk of hyperkalemia. Do not use with diabetic patients who are likely to develop electrolyte imbalances.

Side effects/adverse reactions: Potassium-sparing diuretics may cause severe and potentially fatal hyperkalemia in susceptible patients. Use of spironolactone may be associated with masculinizing effects on females

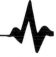

Table 13-4

POTASSIUM-SPARING DIURETICS

Generic name	Trade name	Initial dosage	Maximum per day	Administration
Amiloride	Midamor	5 mg/day	10 mg/day	Oral
Spironolactone	Aldactone	100 mg/day for 5 days	25-200 mg/day in 1 to 4 doses	Oral
Triamterene	Dyrenium	100 mg twice daily after meals	300 mg/day	Oral

NOTE: See manufacturers' guidelines for complete dosage information.

Table 13-5

COMBINATIONS OF THIAZIDE AND POTASSIUM-SPARING DIURETICS

Generic name and dosage	Trade name
Hydrochlorothiazide 25 mg/Amiloride 5 mg	Moduretic
Hydrochlorothiazide 25 mg/Spironolactone 25 mg	Aldactazide 25/25
	Spirozide
Hydrochlorothiazide 50 mg/Spironolactone 50 mg	Aldactazide 50/50
Hydrochlorothiazide 25 mg/Triamterene 50 mg	Dyazide
Hydrochlorothiazide 50 mg/Triamterene 75 mg	Maxide

NOTE: See manufacturers' guidelines for complete dosage information.

and feminizing effects on males as a result of competition with the more potent androgen testosterone.

Pharmacokinetics: Administration with food increases absorption.

Interactions: The half-life of digoxin may be increased by potassium-sparing diuretics. Administration of potassium may result in hyperkalemia.

Nursing considerations: Carefully monitor patients for fluid and electrolyte imbalances, particularly patients receiving digitalis preparations. Instruct the patient that potassium supplements are not to be used.

Combination Diuretic Products

Hydrochlorothiazide is frequently combined with a potassium-sparing diuretic. These products are often more effective than either drug alone. See Table 13-5 for examples of combined products.

IMMUNOSUPPRESSIVE AGENTS

Primary renal disease may stem from immunologic causes, as with lupus erythematosus and acute glomerulonephritis. In these situations immunosuppressive agents have shown some limited benefit. These drugs are primarily used to reduce graft rejection after renal transplantation. The optimum treatment schedules for many agents or drug combinations have yet to be firmly established. A variety of suppression regimens have been used, with increasingly higher graft preservation rates and reduced renal damage.

Antilymphocyte Globulin, Antithymocyte Globulin

Antilymphocyte globulin (ALG) and antithymocyte globulin (Atgam) have been used for many years to reduce transplant rejection. The drugs are prepared from animal serum and depress the primary humoral immune response. The agents' usefulness is limited by their side effects, and their use has decreased with the development of newer agents. The drugs are not ad-

ministered alone, but usually with corticosteroids and other immunosuppressant agents.

Indications: Management of graft rejection in renal transplantation patients or to delay the onset of the first rejection episode. Administered as an adjunct to other therapy.

Usual dosage: *Antilymphocyte globulin* (ALG): 20-30 mg/kg by IV infusion prior to transplantation and for the next three days; 10 mg/kg daily for next 4 weeks; 10 mg/kg every other day for fifth and sixth weeks; then 10 mg/kg every third day during followup. *Antithymocyte globulin* (ATG): 10-30 mg/kg/day by IV infusion. Usually 15 mg/kg is administered daily for 14 days, followed by 15 mg/kg every other day for 14 days.

Precautions/contraindications: The drugs are prepared from animal serum and may precipitate an allergic reaction or anaphylaxis at any time during therapy. Do not administer to patients with a history of reaction to equine gamma globulin preparations or prior reaction to the drug or before sensitivity testing.

Side effects/adverse reactions: Fever, chills, leukopenia, thrombocytopenia, and skin reactions are the most commonly reported adverse effects. Anaphylactic reactions are uncommon but may be life threatening. Serum sickness may occur, as may local reactions at the injection site.

Pharmacokinetics: Not reported.

Interactions: None reported.

Nursing considerations: Infusions should be administered slowly. Follow manufacturer's directions for storage, dilution, and rate of flow. Administer the infusion through a large vein or central vein if possible to reduce the incidence of thrombophlebitis. Carefully assess all patients for signs of allergic reactions. Resuscitation equipment and medications (epinephrine, antihistamines, and corticosteroids) should always be immediately available when administering the drug. Before administration, test patients with an intradermal injection of 0.1 ml of a 1:1,000 dilution of ATG or 1:10 dilution of ALG and a saline control. A localized reaction indicates the need for extreme caution with administration. A systemic reaction to intradermal testing contraindicates systemic administration. Allergic reactions may occur in individuals with negative skin sensitivity tests. Corticosteroids and antihistamines may limit adverse effects. When the drug is used to prevent initial graft rejection, the first dose should be administered within 24 hours of transplantation.

Azathioprine

Azathioprine (Imuran) has been used with considerable success in renal transplantation patients. The drug suppresses T cell function, but the exact mechanism is not known. The drug has a slow onset and a long duration of action, with effects that persist after the drug has been discontinued. Azathioprine has been effective in reducing the incidence of graft rejection, but it has little effect once rejection has been established.

Indications: As an adjunct in preventing rejection of renal allografts. Used in conjunction with corticosteroids and cytotoxic agents. (Also used to treat severe rheumatoid arthritis not responsive to conventional treatment.)

Usual dosage: Initially 3-5 mg/kg/day before transplantation, begun the day of transplantation or several days before transplantation. Maintenance doses are individualized in the 1-3 mg/kg/day range. The drug is administered orally or intravenously in the same doses.

Precautions/contraindications: Contraindicated in hypersensitive patients.

Side effects/adverse reactions: Severe bone marrow depression may occur, usually late in therapy. Azathioprine is carcinogenic in animals and increases the risk of neoplasm in humans. Nausea, vomiting, and other gastrointestinal (GI) disturbance are common, especially during the first months of therapy. Hepatotoxicity has been reported.

Pharmacokinetics: About 30% of the drug is protein bound. Metabolism occurs in erythrocytes and the liver. The drug's effect and duration may vary significantly between individuals. A reduced dose may be used in cases of severe renal dysfunction.

Interactions: Hepatic metabolism of azathioprine is decreased by allopurinol. Doses of azathioprine may be reduced to one third to one fourth of the usual dose.

Nursing considerations: Complete blood counts should be performed weekly during the first month of therapy, twice monthly during the second and third months of therapy, and at least monthly thereafter. The dosage may need to be reduced or the drug stopped completely if severe bone marrow depression occurs. Administration after meals or divided doses may reduce the incidence or severity of GI disturbances. The patient should notify the physician if signs of bleeding or infection occur.

Cyclosporine

Cyclosporine (Sandimmune) is an antibacterial agent related to the polysporin group of antibiotics. Cyclosporine acts against cytotoxic and T-helper cells as they are being sensitized by antigen. Cyclosporine also suppresses the synthesis and secretion of interleukin-2 and inhibits receptor formation on maturing cytotoxic T cells. Administration of cyclosporine at the time of antigen presentation and lymphocyte sensitization is crucial. The drug is administered orally in olive oil or intravenously in polyoxyethylated castor oil.

Indications: Suppression of rejection of bone marrow, kidney, liver, heart, and other allogenic transplants. Generally used in conjunction with adrenal corticosteroids.

Usual dosage: Oral dose is 15 mg/kg/day, first given 4-12 hours before transplantation; after the surgery, this dosage is continued for at least a week, then slowly tapered to a maintenance dose of 5-10 mg/kg/day. The intravenous dose is one third of the oral dose.

Precautions/contraindications: Contraindicated in patients hypersensitive to cyclosporine or polyoxyethylated castor oil (IV administration).

Side effects/adverse reactions: The drug is associated with both nephrotoxicity and hepatotoxicity. Serum creatinine and blood urea nitrogen (BUN) show an increase during therapy and may not necessarily indicate rejection of the transplanted organ. Rapid rises may be treated by reducing the dose. Use of the drug has been associated with an increase in lymphomas.

Hypertension, tremor, hirsutism, and gum hyperplasia may also occur in patients treated with cyclosporine. Since cyclosporine suppresses immune function, patients are at increased risk of infection.

Pharmacokinetics: GI absorption varies considerably. The drug is about 90% protein bound and is distributed primarily outside the blood volume. Blood levels may be monitored, with trough levels of 250-800 ng/ml (whole blood) or 50-300 ng/ml (plasma) associated with minimized side effects and graft rejection. The drug is thoroughly metabolized in the liver through the cytochrome P-450 enzyme system.

Interactions: A variety of drugs alter the pharmacokinetics of cyclosporine, and the drug information sheet should be reviewed before the patient is given any additional drug. Nephrotoxicity is increased when cyclosporine is administered with acyclovir, aminoglycosides, amphotericin B, sulfamethoxazole and/or trimethoprim, nonsteroidal antiinflammatory agents, and melphalan. Convulsions have been reported when cyclosporine is administered with methylprednisolone.

Increased immunosuppression may follow administration with azathioprine, corticosteroids, cyclophosphamide, and verapamil.

Nursing considerations: Renal and hepatic function should be tested and monitored during therapy. The patient should be monitored and evaluated for infection and instructed to notify the physician if fever, sore throat, or other signs of infection develop. To make the oral solution more pleasant, it may be mixed with milk, chocolate milk, or orange juice at room temperature. The drink should be stirred and drunk immediately.

Muromonab-CD3

Muromonab-CD3 (Orthoclone OKT3) is a monoclonal antibody to the T3 antigen of human T cells. The drug blocks T cell function, which plays a major role in renal graft rejection. A rapid decrease in circulating T cells is seen following administration of muromonab.

Indications: Treatment of acute allograft rejection after renal transplantation.

Usual dosage: 5 mg/day for 10 days to 2 weeks. Administered only intravenously.

Precautions/contraindications: Do not administer to patients with fluid overload (evidenced on chest x-ray or weight gain greater than 3% in 1 week). Antibody production develops in most patients, increasing the likelihood of a serious reaction on subsequent courses of treatment.

Side effects/adverse reactions: A large number of patients receiving muromonab experience a temperature elevation, chills, dyspnea, and malaise following drug administration. Potentially fatal pulmonary edema has been reported in patients with fluid overload at the start of treatment.

Pharmacokinetics: Serum levels stabilized after the third day of treatment, averaging 0.9 μg/ml.

Interactions: None reported.

Nursing considerations: Muromonab is administered only intravenously and should be given as a bolus in less than 1 minute; it should not be administered by IV infusion. Patients should have a clear chest x-ray within 24 hours before the first dose. Respiratory function should be closely monitored after the initial dose. To decrease the incidence of adverse reactions, adrenal corticosteroids may be given before and after administration. Acetaminophen and antihistamines may be used to treat reactions. Adverse effects generally decrease on successive days of treatment.

Chlorambucil and Cyclophosphamide

Chlorambucil and cyclophosphamide are nitrogen mustards used most commonly as chemotherapeutic agents in the treatment of neoplasms. They are also used in the treatment of certain renal disorders.

Chlorambucil

With the exception of bone marrow depression, chlorambucil (Leukeran) is relatively free of toxicity.

Indications: Chlorambucil has been used in combination with corticosteroids in the treatment of idiopathic membranous nephropathy.

Usual dosage: 0.1-0.2 mg/kg/day every other month, alternating with corticosteroids for 6 months.

Precautions/contraindications: Contraindicated in hypersensitive patients.

Side effects/adverse reactions: Bone marrow depression, which is usually reversible when the drug is discontinued, is the most significant adverse effect. A variety of other less common adverse effects may occur, including GI disturbances, hepatotoxicity, pulmonary fibrosis, bronchopulmonary dysplasia, male sterility, drug fever, skin reactions, and CNS disturbances. Chlorambucil may be carcinogenic.

Pharmacokinetics: GI absorption is rapid and complete, with a high degree of plasma protein binding. Metabolism occurs in the liver.

Interactions: None reported.

Nursing considerations: Monitor the patient for adverse effects. Perform complete blood counts periodically during therapy. Instruct the patient to report signs of bleeding, infection, or other adverse effects to the physician.

Cyclophosphamide

Cyclophosphamide (Cytoxan, Neosar) has immunosuppressive effects in addition to its antineoplastic action.

Indications: Biopsy proven "minimal change" nephrotic syndrome especially in children, who did not respond satisfactorily to corticosteroids.

Usual dosage: 2.5-3 mg/kg/day in oral form for up to 60-90 days.

Precautions/contraindications: Administration beyond 60-90 days increases the incidence of male sterility. Contraindicated in hypersensitive patients.

Side effects/adverse reactions: Bone marrow suppression is the most severe and common adverse effect. The adverse effects are usually reversible if the drug is discontinued. A significant number of patients may develop acute hemorrhagic cystitis. Skin disturbances, alopecia, and GI disturbances frequently occur. Cardiac and pulmonary toxicity are less common adverse effects. Use of the drug may lead to sterility in both males and females or may be carcinogenic. Most adverse effects are reversible with discontinuance of the drug.

Pharmacokinetics: Well absorbed from the GI tract. Low protein binding with metabolism in the liver.

Interactions: Digoxin serum levels may be increased. Leukopenia may be prolonged by thiazide diuretics. The drug half-life is increased by chloramphenicol.

Nursing considerations: Monitor complete blood counts and renal function during therapy. Instruct the patient to report signs of bleeding, infection, or other adverse effects to the physician.

Corticosteroids

Even though their precise mechanism of action is not known, corticosteroids have been used for many years to treat inflammation. Naturally occurring glucocorticoids, such as cortisol and cortisone, have effects also associated with the mineralocorticoids (i.e., sodium retention, potassium excretion, hypertension). The development of synthetic glucocorticoids has lead to agents with enhanced antiinflammatory effects with reduced mineralocorticoid effects. The qualitative differences among the synthetic antiinflammatory steroids is minimal; differences involve the potency of the antiinflammatory effects and their duration of action.

Corticosteroids are used in the treatment of nephrotic syndrome and for their antiinflammatory and immunosuppressant effects in reducing graft rejection.

Usual dose: The use, dosage, and administration of corticosteroids vary widely.

Precautions/contraindications: Use with caution in patients with peptic ulcer, heart disease, or hypertension with CHF, infections, psychoses, diabetes, osteoporosis, glaucoma, or herpes infection.

Side effects/adverse reactions: Side effects are uncommon with short-term therapy (less than 1 week) but increase with the duration of therapy. Undesirable effects that may occur during prolonged systemic use at high doses include truncal obesity and cushingoid features, hyperglycemia, sodium retention with edema, hypertension, weight gain, muscle wasting, acne, hypokalemia, peptic ulcers, osteoporosis, increased intraocular pressure, cataract development, psychosis, and exacerbation of infections. Suppression of adrenal function also occurs when these drugs are administered over a long period.

Pharmacokinetics: *Onset of action:* Slow. *Plasma half-life:* Prednisone, 60 min; methylprednisolone, 78-188 min. *Route of elimination:* Metabolized in the liver, with renal excretion.

Interactions: The patient's need for insulin or hypoglycemic agents may increase. Phenytoin, phenobarbital, rifampin, and possibly ephedrine may increase metabolism of corticosteroids and reduce the effectiveness of a given dose. Oral contraceptives may inhibit corticosteroid metabolism.

Nursing considerations: Monitor all patients for development of adverse effects. Patients having long-term therapy must have the drug dose slowly tapered to avoid adrenal insufficiency (Cushing's syndrome). Assess all patients for signs of adrenal insufficiency during withdrawal of systemic therapy. During periods of stress, patients recently withdrawn from systemic steroids should have treatment resumed.

PHOSPHATE-BINDING AGENTS

Aluminum carbonate (Basaljel) and aluminum hydroxide (Alu-cap, Dialume, Amphojel, Alternagel) are antacids that are used for their phosphate-binding capabilities in the treatment of hyperphosphatemia associated with chronic renal failure. The antacids may also be used to reduce phosphate absorption and, hopefully, stone formation in patients with recurrent phosphate urinary stones. Antacids containing aluminum combine with ingested phosphates in the intestine to form insoluble complexes that are excreted in the feces. Therapy is usually combined with a low-phosphate diet. The antacid is administered with meals, in a 30-40 ml dose of aluminum hydroxide or aluminum carbonate suspension. Ideally the dose should be in proportion to the phosphate content of the meal. Of the two antacids, aluminum carbonate has more phosphate-binding capability. These antacids are constipating and should be administered with a stool softener. With ingestion of the large amounts of aluminum contained in the suspensions, there is a risk of increased aluminum absorption leading to osteomalacia or neurotoxicity.

Calcium acetate (Phos-Ex) is a non–aluminum containing phosphate binder used in the treatment of the hyperphosphatemia of renal disease. Given with meals, the calcium combines with dietary phosphate and is excreted in the feces. It is not constipating. The usual dose is 2 tablets (667 mg each) with meals, gradually increasing to 3 or 4 tablets with each meal. The only side effects reported are increased calcium levels and nausea.

The use of calcium acetate is contraindicated in patients with hypercalcemia. Since calcium acetate may increase serum calcium levels, do not give additional calcium. Consider the calcium in the diet and in dialysate, if appropriate. Monitor serum calcium and phosphate levels; the Ca × P product should not exceed 66. Do not use with patients receiving digoxin because cardiac arrhythmias may be precipitated.

ANTIINFECTIVE AGENTS

Many antibiotics require some adjustments (either reduced frequency or dosage) when administered to patients with severely reduced renal function. The exact dosages are based on the degree of renal excretion of the drug, the location and type of infecting organism (determines tissue levels needed), and the degree of renal function (based on creatinine clearance). When dialysis patients are receiving antibiotics, the drugs are most often administered after dialysis, since dialysis affects the serum level of most antibiotics. Refer to the package insert and the manufacturer's recommendations when determining antibiotic doses for patients with decreased renal function.

Penicillins

Penicillins are the most widely effective and widely used antibiotics. Penicillins and cephalosporins are two large groups of antibiotic drugs that share similar properties. These drugs are referred to as beta-lactam drugs. Antibiotics in this class exert their effect by inhibiting cell wall synthesis. Penicillin G, the prototype penicillin, was first discovered in 1929. The penicillins differ significantly in degree of inactivation by gastric acids, protein binding, inactivation by penicillinase, and spectrum of antimicrobial activity.

Resistance to many of the penicillins may develop if organisms produce an enzyme, beta-lactamase (also called penicillinase), that inactivates some penicillins by breaking the beta-lactam ring in their structure. Penicillins resistant to these enzymes are called "penicillinase resistant." Combinations of a penicillin with a beta-lactamase inhibitor are available. The combination is thought to increase the effectiveness of penicillin by inhibiting bacterial beta-lactamase.

The amidinopenicillins are a new group of penicillins, of which amdinocillin is the prototype. Because this drug binds with different receptors than those used by other penicillins, it may be synergistic with other penicillins.

Indications: Infections caused by penicillin-sensitive bacteria.

Usual dosage: Varies (see Table 13-6). The dosage of most penicillins must be reduced in patients with decreased renal function. Hemodialysis affects the serum level of most penicillins but not of cloxacillin. Peritoneal dialysis affects the blood level of most penicillins but not of methicillin or cloxacillin.

Precautions/contraindications: All penicillins are cross-sensitizing (a patient allergic to any one penicillin is allergic to all penicillins) and cross-reacting.

Side effects/adverse reactions: The incidence of allergic reactions to the penicillins has been estimated to be as high as 5% to 10% in adults. Original sensitizing exposure may come from exposure to environmental mold and dermatophytes living on the skin that can produce penicillin-like molecules. Another source of exposure is penicillin in the milk of cows being treated for mastitis. Allergic reactions may be immediate (pruritus, urticaria, asthma, rhinitis, laryngeal edema, anaphylaxis), intermediate (rashes and fever), or delayed, even after the antibiotic is stopped (serum sickness,

rashes, thrombocytopenia, anemias). Anaphylactic reactions have an estimated incidence of 0.01% to 0.04% and are most common after parenteral therapy.

Although irritating to tissues, penicillins are not highly toxic. Large doses may produce GI upset, local pain may accompany intramuscular injections, and sclerosing phlebitis may follow intravenous administration. Although infrequent, interstitial nephritis and nephropathy have been associated with high doses of penicillin administered parenterally. High doses of ticarcillin, carbenicillin, mezlocillin, piperacillin, azlocillin, or nafcillin have been reported to cause bleeding abnormalities.

Many penicillins have a high sodium content, which may lead to electrolyte imbalances when high doses of the drug are administered, particularly in cases of reduced renal function. Sodium penicillin G contains 2 mEq of sodium per 1 million units (1 mEq sodium = 23 mg), and potassium penicillin G contains 1.7 mEq of potassium per 1 million units. Hypokalemia has been reported in patients receiving azlocillin, mezlocillin, ticarcillin, piperacillin, and carbenicillin.

Ampicillin frequently causes skin rashes, some of which are not related to allergy.

Bone marrow depression with granulocytopenia or interstitial nephritis may occur with the penicillinase-resistant penicillins.

Pharmacokinetics: Penicillins are primarily excreted through the kidneys. Nafcillin is least dependent on renal excretion, with about 80% of a dose excreted in the bile. Penicillin is also excreted in saliva and milk in roughly 3% to 15% of serum levels. Penicillin G and several other penicillin drugs may be either partially or totally inactivated by gastric acids with a pH of 2 or less. Absorption of most penicillins is affected by food.

Penicillins may be formulated to have a prolonged action following intramuscular administration. Procaine or benzathine salts are used for intramuscular administration to maintain effective serum concentrations for up to 4 weeks as the result of slow, prolonged absorption from the injection site.

Interactions: Administration of probenecid blocks renal excretion of penicillin and prolongs blood levels. Probenecid may be administered with the penicillin for this effect. Increased incidences of breakthrough bleeding and pregnancy have been reported following the use of some penicillins in patients using oral contraceptives.

Nursing considerations: Penicillins (except amoxicillin and penicillin V) should not be administered at meal times but at least 1 hour before meals or 1 to 3 hours after meals to minimize protein binding or inactivation by gastric acid. All patients should be monitored closely for signs of immediate or delayed allergic reaction.

Table 13-6

PENICILLINS

Generic name	Trade name	Dosage	Administration
Penicillin G	Pentids	200,000-400,000 U q 6-8 h	Oral
Penicillin G	Pfizerpen	2-50 million U/day in 2 divided doses	IM, IV
Procaine penicillin G	Duracillin	600,000-1.2 million U/day in 2 divided doses	IM
Penicillin V	Pen-Vee K, SK Penicillin VK, V-Cillin K	200,000-400,000 U q 6-8 h	Oral
Penicillinase resistant			
Methicillin	Staphcillin, Dimocillin	4-12 g/day in 4-6 divided doses	IM, IV
Nafcillin	Unipen, Nafcil, Nallpen	1-6 g/day in 4-6 divided doses	Oral
		2-12 g/day in 4-6 divided doses	IM, IV
Oxacillin	Prostaphlin, Bactocill	1-6 g/day in 4-6 divided doses	Oral
		1-12 g/day in 4-6 divided doses	IM, IV
Cloxacillin	Cloxapen, Tegopen	1-4 g/day in 4 divided doses	Oral
Dicloxacillin	Dynapen, Pathocil	0.5-1.0 g/day in 4 divided doses	Oral
Ampicillins			
Ampicillin	Ampicill, Omnipen, Polycillin, Totacillin	1-4 g/day in 4 divided doses	Oral
		1-12 g/day in 4-8 divided doses	IM, IV
Bacampicillin	Spectrobid	400 mg-1.6 g q 12 h	Oral
Amoxicillin	Amoxil, Larotid, Polymox, Trimox	250-500 mg q 8 h	Oral
Cyclacillin	Cyclapen	250-500 mg q 6 h	Oral
Extended spectrum			
Carbenicillin	Geopen, Pyopen	250-500 mg/kg/day in divided doses	IM, IV
Carbenicillin indanyl	Geocillin	382-764 mg q6h	Oral
Ticarcillin	Ticar	150-300 mg/kg/day in 3-6 divided doses	IM, IV
Mezlocillin	Mezlin	100-300 mg/kg/day in 4-6 divided doses	IM, IV
Piperacillin	Pipracil	8-18 g/day in 2-6 divided doses	IM, IV
Azlocillin	Azlin	100-350 mg/kg/day in 4-6 divided doses	IV
Amidinopenicillins			
Amdinocillin	Coactin	10 mg/kg/day in 4-6 divided doses	IM, IV
Combined penicillin/beta-lactamase inhibitors			
Amoxicillin/clavulanic acid	Augmentin	250 or 500 mg/125 mg q 8 h	Oral
Ticarcillin/clavulanic acid	Timentin	3g/100 mg q 4-8 h	IV
Ampicillin/sulbactam	Unasyn	1-2 g/0.5-1 g q 6 h	IM, IV

Dosage, interval, or both may need to be altered with reduced renal function. See manufacturers' guidelines for complete dosage information.

When administering parenteral penicillins, emergency drugs for treating anaphylaxis should be immediately available. Caution women using oral contraceptives to use an alternate method of birth control during antibiotic therapy. Monitor patients at risk for electrolyte imbalance for signs of potassium imbalance, sodium imbalance, or water retention.

Cephalosporins

The cephalosporins are beta-lactams similar to penicillins. They are bactericidal, interfering with cell wall synthesis. Cephalosporin antibiotics are classified as first-, second-, or third-generation forms. The terminology, which was developed for marketing, does not always follow the chronologic development of the drugs, but it does follow their spectrum of antibacterial activity. Progressing through first-, second-, and third-generation cephalosporins, the effectiveness against gram-negative organisms generally increases, whereas the effectiveness against gram-positive organisms decreases.

Indications: Treatment of cephalosporin-sensitive bacterial infections; surgical prophylaxis.

Usual dosage: Varies (see Table 13-7). The dosage of most cephalosporins must be reduced for patients with diminished renal function. Hemodialysis and peritoneal dialysis probably affect the serum levels of most cephalosporins.

Precautions/contraindications: Cross-sensitivity with the penicillins has been reported but is not always seen.

Side effects/adverse reactions: Allergic reactions

Table 13-7

CEPHALOSPORINS

Generic name	Trade name	Dosage range	Administration
First generation			
Cephalothin	Keflin	0.5-2 g q 4-6 h	IM, IV
Cefazolin	Ancef, Kefzol, Zolicef	0.25-1.5 g q 6-8 h	IM, IV
Cephapirin	Cefadyl	0.5-2 g q 4-6 h	IM, IV
Cephradine	Anspor, Velosef	250 mg-1 g q 6-12 h	Oral
		500 mg-1 g q 6 h	IM, IV
Cephalexin	Keflet, Keflex, Keftab	250-500 mg q 6-12 h	Oral
Cefadroxil	Duricef, Ultracef	1-2 g/day q 12-24 h	Oral
Second generation			
Cefamandole	Mandol	0.5-1 g q 4-8 h	IM, IV
Cefuroxime	Ceftin	250-500 mg 2 times/day	Oral
	Kefurox, Zinacef	0.75-1.5 g q 8 h	IM, IV
Cefonicid	Monocid	1 g q 24 h	IM, IV
Cefoxitin	Mefoxin	1-2 g q 6-8 h	IM, IV
Cefaclor	Ceclor	250-500 mg q 8 h	Oral
Cefotetan	Cefotan	1-2 g q 12 h	IM, IV
Ceforanide	Precef	0.5-1 g q 12 h	IM, IV
Cefmetazole	Zefazone	2 g q 6-12 h	IV
Third generation			
Cefotaxime	Claforan	1-2 g/day q 6-8 h	IM, IV
Ceftriaxone	Rocephin	1-2 g/day in 1 or 2 doses	IM, IV
Moxalactam	Moxam	1-4 g/day q 8-12 h	IM, IV
Cefoperazone	Cefobid	1-2 g q 12 h	IM, IV
Ceftizoxime	Cefizox	0.5-2 g q 8-12 h	IM, IV
Ceftazidime	Fortaz, Tazidime	0.5-2 g q 8-12 h	IM, IV
Cefixime	Suprax	400 mg/day	Oral

Dosage, interval, or both may need to be altered with reduced renal function. See manufacturers' guidelines for complete dosage information.

and tissue irritations are similar in nature and incidence to those with penicillins. Renal toxicity has been reported with some of the early cephalosporins, especially when used with an aminoglycoside antibiotic.

Pharmacokinetics: Most of the cephalosporins are poorly absorbed from the GI tract, and therefore most are administered parenterally. Most cephalosporins are excreted primarily by the kidneys. Cefoperazone in excreted primarily in the bile. Food may increase or decrease absorption, depending on which oral cephalosporin is used.

Interactions: The nephrotoxicity of aminoglycosides may be potentiated. Oral anticoagulants may have an increased effect. Nausea and vomiting may occur if alcohol is consumed while the drug is in the body.

Nursing considerations: See Penicillins (page 202).

Aminoglycosides

The aminoglycoside antibiotics are effective against a wide range of bacteria, but their toxicity limits their use primarily to treatment of serious gram-negative infections. The aminoglycosides exert their bactericidal effects by interfering with protein synthesis. Oral forms of aminoglycosides are not significantly absorbed and are used to suppress GI flora in preparation for abdominal surgery or for reducing ammonia-forming bacteria in the treatment of hepatic coma.

Indications: Parenteral administration is used to treat gram-negative infections. Streptomycin is used as an antitubercular drug. Oral forms are used to suppress GI flora in preparation for abdominal surgery or to reduce ammonia-forming bacteria in the treatment of hepatic coma. Paromomycin is used in the treatment of intestinal amebiasis.

Usual dosage: Varies (see Table 13-8). Reduced dosage is necessary for patients with reduced renal function. The aminoglycosides are affected by both hemodialysis and peritoneal dialysis. Because of these drugs' high potential for nephrotoxicity, therapy in patients with significant renal impairment must be guided by serum levels, with close monitoring of renal function.

Precautions/contraindications: Not used for long-term therapy because of the high incidence of ototoxicity and nephrotoxicity. Dehydration and advanced age increase the risk of toxicity. These drugs may aggravate muscle weakness, especially in patients with neuromuscular disorders such as myasthenia gravis.

Side effects/adverse reactions: Aminoglycosides are associated with nephrotoxicity and ototoxicity even at conventional doses. Renal damage may be manifested by decreased creatinine clearance, cells or casts in urine, oliguria, proteinuria, or increased serum blood urea nitrogen or creatinine. The renal damage may be reversible. The drugs are toxic to the eighth cranial nerve, causing both auditory and vestibular damage. The damage may appear as high-frequency hearing loss, tinnitus, or vertigo. Deafness may develop several weeks after administration of the drug has been stopped, and it may be irreversible. High doses may be neurotoxic and may have a neuromuscular blocking effect.

Pharmacokinetics: Oral forms are not significantly absorbed, whereas absorption is rapid and complete following intramuscular administration. The unchanged drug is excreted through the kidneys, and excretion is markedly decreased with decreased renal function.

Interactions: The potential for ototoxicity or nephrotoxicity is greater when aminoglycosides are adminis-

Table 13-8

AMINOGLYCOSIDES

Generic name	Trade name	Dosage range*	Administration
Amikacin	Amikin	15 mg/kg/day in 2-3 doses	IM, IV
Gentamicin	Garamycin	3-5 mg/kg q 8 h	IM, IV
Kanamycin	Kantrex, Klebcil	15 mg/kg/day in 2-3 doses	IM
		4-12 g/day	Oral
Neomycin	Mycifradin, Neobiotic	15 mg/kg/day in 4 doses	IM
		3-12 g/day in 4 doses	Oral
Netilmicin	Neo-IM, Netromycin	3-6.5 mg/kg/day in 3-4 doses	IM, IV
Paromomycin	Humatin	25-35 mg/kg/day in 8 doses	Oral
Streptomycin		1-4 g/day in 2-4 doses	IM
Tobramycin*	Nebcin	3-5 mg/kg q 8 h	IM, IV

Dosage, interval, or both may need to be altered with reduced renal function. See manufacturers' guidelines for complete dosage information.

tered with other aminoglycosides, parenteral forms of amphotericin B, bumetanide, cephalosporins, cyclosporine, ethacrynic acid, furosemide, and vancomycin.

Nursing considerations: Dosage should be reduced in elderly patients or patients with reduced renal function. Renal function, hearing, and vestibular function should be assessed before and during high-dose or long-term therapy (longer than 10 days). Intravenous administration should be accomplished over a period of 30 to 60 minutes to reduce the possibility of toxic serum levels. Patients should be well hydrated and should be instructed to report any hearing loss, tinnitus, or dizziness. Peak and trough serum levels should be monitored.

Fluoroquinolones

Ciprofloxacin and norfloxacin are synthetic, broad-spectrum antibacterial agents. They work through inhibition of protein synthesis.

Indications: Because of its poor bioavailability and low serum concentrations, norfloxacin is approved only for treatment of urinary tract infections. Ciprofloxacin is indicated for both urinary and systemic infections.

Usual dosage: Norfloxacin (Noroxin), 400 mg q 12 hr; ciprofloxacin (Cipro), 250-750 mg q 12 hr. Both drugs are administered only orally.

Precautions/contraindications: Use with caution in patients with known or suspected central nervous system (CNS) disorders or with a predisposition to seizures. The dosage may need to be reduced in patients with diminished renal function.

Side effects/adverse reactions: CNS stimulation, including tremors, restlessness, light-headedness, and seizures may occur with ciprofloxacin. Nausea, vomiting, or diarrhea may occur with either drug.

Pharmacokinetics: Both drugs are absorbed well and excreted primarily through the kidneys; they have an increased half-life if the patient has decreased renal function. Food may decrease the absorption of norfloxacin. Absorption of ciprofloxacin is delayed if food is present in the stomach, but overall absorption is not altered.

Interactions: Antacids containing magnesium or aluminum hydroxide may interfere with absorption of ciprofloxacin. Theophylline levels may be increased, because theophylline clearance is reduced in patients taking fluoroquinolones.

Nursing considerations: Norfloxacin tablets should be taken 1 hour before or 2 hours after meals. Ciprofloxacin may be taken with or without meals. Patients should be well hydrated. Patients taking theophylline should be monitored for signs of toxic effects, and their serum theophylline levels should be monitored.

Sulfonamides and Trimethoprim
Sulfonamides

The sulfonamides are bacteriostatic drugs. They competitively antagonize paraaminobenzoic acid (PABA), which is essential for folic acid synthesis. Microorganisms that require endogenous folic acid are therefore susceptible to the sulfonamides.

Indications: The sulfonamides have a broad spectrum of activity; however, they are most often used to treat urinary tract infections or in topical preparations.

Usual dosage: Varies (see Tables 13-9 and 13-10).

Table 13-9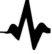

SULFONAMIDES FOR SYSTEMIC USE

Generic name	Trade name	Dosage	Administration
Sulfacytine	Renoquid	500 mg initially, then 250 mg q 4 h for 10 days	Oral
Sulfadiazine	Microsulfon	2-4 g initially, then 2-4 g/day in 3-6 equal doses	Oral
Sulfamethizole	Proklar	0.5-1 g in 3-4 doses daily (total 1.5-4 g)	Oral
Sulfamethoxazole	Gantanol Gamazole	2 g initially then 1 g 2 or 3 times/day	Oral
Sulfapyridine		500 mg 4 times/day	Oral
Sulfasalazine	Azaline Azulfidine	3-4 g/day initially, then 2 g/day in 4 equal doses	Oral
Sulfisoxazole	Gantrisin Gulfasin	2-4 g/day initially, then 4-8 g/day in 4-6 equal doses	Oral

Dose and/or interval may need to be altered with reduced renal function. See manufacturers' guidelines for complete dosage information.

Precautions/contraindications: In patients with porphyria, sulfonamides may precipitate an attack. Photosensitivity can occur.

Side effects/adverse reactions: Nausea, vomiting, abdominal pain, photosensitivity, rashes, pruritus, and exfoliative dermatitis can occur. Cross-sensitivity can occur in patients sensitive to carbonic anhydrase inhibitors, thiazides, furosemide, bumetanide, and the sulfonylurea hypoglycemic agents. Sulfonamides can cause blood dyscrasias, including anemia, granulocytopenia, and thrombocytopenia. The drugs also can precipitate in the urine, causing crystalluria, hematuria, or obstruction.

Pharmacokinetics: Sulfonamides are readily absorbed from the GI tract and excreted mainly through the kidneys.

Interactions: Sulfonamides may displace highly protein bound drugs (e.g., oral anticoagulants, anticonvulsants, and oral antidiabetic agents) from protein binding sites, resulting in higher serum levels and increased effects. The potential for toxic effects is increased when sulfonamides are administered with hepatotoxic or bone marrow-suppressing drugs.

Nursing considerations: Instruct the patient to take each dose on an empty stomach with a large glass of water. If GI upset occurs, instruct the patient to take the drug with food. Urinary solubility depends on pH. Alkalinization of the urine and a high urine output help prevent precipitation in the urine. Caution patients to avoid or minimize exposure to sunlight and to use sunscreens when outside.

Trimethoprim

Trimethoprim blocks the production of folic acid at a site different than that of the sulfonamides.

Indications: Treatment of urinary tract infections.

Usual dosage: 100 mg q 12h or 200 mg/day.

Precautions/contraindications: Use with caution in patients with renal or hepatic impairment.

Side effects/adverse reactions: Rashes, pruritus, exfoliative dermatitis, and GI disturbances can occur. In rare cases trimethoprim causes bone marrow depression, usually associated with large doses or prolonged administration.

Pharmacokinetics: Trimethoprim is well absorbed after oral administration; primary excretion is through the kidneys.

Interactions: Trimethoprim may augment the effect of phenytoin as a result of inhibition of metabolism.

Nursing considerations: The tablets should be protected from light.

Trimethoprim-sulfamethoxazole

The combination of trimethoprim and sulfamethoxazole results in a double block of folate synthesis; this provides a synergistic effect with increased activity and a wider antibacterial spectrum. The combination is used primarily to treat urinary tract infections. (See individual drugs for profile and nursing considerations.) The intravenous form should be administered over 60 to 90 minutes and must be diluted and used within 2 hours of mixing.

Urinary Antibacterial Drugs

Cinoxacin

Cinoxacin (Cinobac) is a synthetic, organic acid related to nalidixic acid, which inhibits replication of bacterial DNA.

Indications: Treatment of urinary tract infections caused by susceptible organisms.

Table 13-10

SULFONAMIDES IN FIXED COMBINATIONS FOR SYSTEMIC USE

Generic name and drug amount	Trade names	Administration
Sulfamethoxazole 400 or 800 mg with trimethoprim 80 or 160 mg also known generically as co-trimoxazole	Septra, Bactrim Septra IV, Bactrim IV	Oral IV
Sulfadiazine 167 mg, sulfamerazine 167 mg, and sulfamethazine 167 mg	Neotrizine	Oral
Sulfamethizole 250 or 500 mg and phenazopyridine 100 mg	Azo-Gantanol	Oral
Sulfamethizole 250 mg, phenazopyridine 50 mg, and oxytetracycline 250 mg	Urobiotic	Oral
Sulfisoxazole 500 mg and phenazopyridine 50 mg	Azo-Gantrisin	Oral

Dose and/or interval may need to be altered with reduced renal function. See manufacturers' guidelines for complete dosage information.

Table 13-11

URINARY ANTIBACTERIALS*

Generic name	Trade name	Dosage	Administration
Cinoxacin	Cinobac	250 mg q6h or 500 mg twice daily for 7-14 days	Oral
Methenamine	Hexamine	1 g 4 times/day after meals and at bedtime	Oral
Nalidixic acid	NegGram	1 g 4 times/day for 7-14 days	Oral
Nitrofurantoin	Furadantin	50-100 mg 4 times/day for 7 days or more	Oral

Do not use with reduced renal function. Note: See manufacturers' guidelines for complete dosage information.

Usual dosage: Varies (see Table 13-11)

Precautions/contraindications: Toxicity may occur in patients with reduced renal function as a result of decreased renal excretion and increased serum levels.

Side effects/adverse reactions: The most common side effects involve GI or genitourinary (GU) disturbances, including nausea, vomiting, diarrhea, abdominal cramps, and perineal burning.

Pharmacokinetics: Cinoxacin is completely absorbed after oral administration. The drug is partly metabolized in the liver, and the metabolites and remaining active drug are excreted in the urine.

Interactions: Not fully established.

Nursing considerations: Caution the patient that the drug may cause dizziness, or the eyes may be more sensitive to light.

Methenamine

Methenamine (Hexamine, Hiprex, Mandelamine, others) is hydrolyzed to ammonia and formaldehyde, which is bactericidal. The drug does not release formaldehyde in the serum. Methenamine is available as acid salts (mandelate and hippurate) to promote a low urinary pH.

Indications: Suppression or elimination of bacterial urinary tract infections.

Usual dosage: Varies (see Table 13-11)

Precautions/contraindications: Do not use methenamine with severe renal failure or dehydration. It also should not be given to patients with liver disease, since the drug promotes production of ammonia.

Side effects/adverse reactions: Large doses can irritate the bladder. Other adverse effects include GI symptoms, stomatitis, and rashes.

Pharmacokinetics: Methenamine and related salts are readily absorbed from the GI tract, with up to 25% subject to hepatic metabolism. The generation of urinary formaldehyde depends on urinary pH, volume, and how long urine is retained in the bladder.

Interactions: Drugs that increase urine pH (bicarbonate, acetazolamide) will reduce effectiveness.

Nursing considerations: Administer methenamine with food to minimize GI upset, and encourage fluids to ensure adequate urine flow. Have the patient avoid or limit alkalinizing foods such as citrus fruits and milk products.

Nalidixic acid

Nalidixic acid (NegGram) is similar to cinoxacin but may produce more GI effects. (See the discussion of cinoxacin for a more detailed presentation.)

Nitrofurantoin

Nitrofurantoin (Furadantin) interferes with bacterial carbohydrate metabolism and may also disrupt cell wall synthesis. The action of nitrofurantoin is increased in an acid pH.

Indications: Treatment of urinary tract infections of susceptible bacteria.

Usual dosage: Varies (see Table 13-11)

Precautions/contraindications: Renal impairment (creatinine clearance less than 40 ml/min), anuria, or oliguria reduces the effectiveness of treatment and greatly increases toxicity.

Side effects/adverse reactions: Fever, rash, eosinophilia, and pulmonary infiltrates can occur. Pulmonary reactions may be acute or chronic and are manifested by dyspnea, chest pain, cough, fever, and chills. The pulmonary damage may be reversible or permanent. Hemolysis can occur in patients with a glucose 6-phosphate dehydrogenase (G6PD) deficiency.

Pharmacokinetics: Nitrofurantoin is well absorbed after oral administration. When the drug is administered with meals, absorption is enhanced. Nitrofurantoin and its metabolites are excreted into the urine, where therapeutic levels are achieved. Serum and tissue levels do not reach therapeutic levels with oral administration in patients with normal renal function.

Interactions: Probenecid can reduce renal clearance and increase serum levels, possibly to toxic levels.

Nursing considerations: Administer nitrofurantoin with meals to improve absorption and minimize GI disturbances. Monitor the patient for signs of pulmonary changes, and instruct him to report any symptoms to the physician.

ERYTHROCYTE-STIMULATING HORMONE
Recombinant human erythropoietin

Erythropoietin is an endogenous hormone produced primarily by the kidneys that promotes the production of red blood cells (erythrocytes). A biosynthetic form of the hormone is available for use in treating anemia secondary to reduced renal production of erythropoietin in patients with chronic renal failure. The biosynthetic form, recombinant human erythropoietin (Epogen), is produced through the use of recombinant DNA techniques and is identical to the endogenous hormone. Due to the length of time required for red blood cells to develop, an increase in hematocrit is usually not seen until 2 weeks after therapy is begun. The rate of increase depends on the dosage, but nearly all patients have a significant increase in hematocrit after 2 months of therapy.

Indications: Treatment of anemia secondary to chronic renal failure.

Usual dosage: Therapy is begun with an intravenous or subcutaneous dose of 50-100 U/kg three times a week. Once the target range is reached, (usually a hematocrit of 30% to 33%) or the hematocrit increases more than 4% in a 2-week period, a maintenance dose is administered. Maintenance doses are individualized; often doses of 25-50 U/kg three times a week are needed.

Precautions/contraindications: Caution should be used when administering recombinant human erythropoietin to hypertensive patients, since the drug may increase blood pressure. The drug is contraindicated in patients allergic to human albumin. Assess patient's iron stores before and during course of therapy.

Side effects/adverse reactions: An increase in blood pressure may be seen during therapy. Skin reactions have been reported but are not common. Polycythemia may occur if the dosage is not properly adjusted.

Pharmacokinetics: Therapeutic levels are maintained for at least 24 hours after intravenous administration. The drug's half-life does not appear to be affected by dialysis.

Interactions: None reported; however, recombinant human erythropoietin should be administered separately from other drugs.

Nursing considerations: Recombinant human erythropoietin is not used for immediate correction of anemia. It may take several weeks to see the response to a dosage adjustment. Supplemental iron may be needed if a clinical response is not seen within several weeks, the patient should be evaluated for other causes of anemia. The drug preparation contains no preservatives, and the vial should be used only once. *Do not shake* the preparation, since shaking may denature the drug and inactivate it.

ANTILITHIC DRUGS

A variety of drugs are used to reduce the formation of stones in the urinary tract. Antacids containing aluminum bind with gastrointestinal phosphate to form insoluble salts, which are then excreted. These antacids are used to reduce phosphate absorption in the intestine in patients with recurrent phosphate urinary stones and to treat hyperphosphatemia associated with renal failure.

Thiazide diuretics have been used to decrease calcium excretion and reduce the risk of calcium precipitation in the urinary tract. Cellulose sodium phosphate (Calcibind) is a binding agent useful in reducing calcium absorption in the GI tract. The drug is used to treat stone formation associated with absorptive hypercalciuria. Stone formation associated with increased uric acid levels may be treated with the uricosuric agent allopurinol (Zyloprim). Potassium citrate or bicarbonate, or sodium citrate or bicarbonate may be administered to promote alkaline urine, which reduces precipitation and formation of uric acid and cystine calculi.

Appendix: Nutrition in Renal Disease

GOALS

To achieve and maintain optimum nutrition
To minimize metabolic disorders and related symptoms
To slow progression of the disease
To delay the need for dialysis

Diet control is a major component of treatment in renal dysfunction. When to begin and what modifications to make are important medical decisions. Significant factors include the level of residual renal function, the use of dialysis, and other conditions such as diabetes mellitus. Even after a renal transplant the individual usually is required to modify his diet because of the side effects of immunosuppressive drugs.

GUIDES TO PROVIDING ADEQUATE NUTRITION

- Assess nutritional needs; consider treatment program
- Assess social factors/limitations
- Assess educational needs
- Individualize diet plan
- Provide patient/family education and encouragement
- Monitor nutritional outcomes
- Modify plan and intervene as needed

Diet-teaching techniques used by the health team are vital to meeting the educational needs of patients and families and to solve problems in compliance. It is important to identify suboptimal intake before deficiency occurs. Eating habits, loss of appetite, diet restrictions, and losses during dialysis may result in undernutrition. The use of exchange diets similar to those long in use for diabetic patients has facilitated learning and adjusting to the diet requirements. Other alternatives are to use lists of foods allowed, not allowed, and "free" foods; or tables listing composition of common foods that permit counting up the amounts of specific nutrients consumed.

Factors that must be controlled in renal disease are fluids, sodium, potassium, proteins, and calories. Vitamin and mineral additions must be considered at the same time. Other substances such as calcium, oxalate, and purines may be controlled when they cause renal calculi.

FLUIDS (WATER)

Function: To maintain body's water composition. Water contributes to (1) structure and form of body (turgor), (2) aqueous environment for cell metabolism, and (3) stable body temperature.

Excess	Deficit
Fluid overload as evidenced by weight gain, edema, dyspnea, and hypertension.	Dehydration causing hypotension, decreased GFR, and decreased ability to excrete the solute load.

Desirable amount: The amounts required depend on solutes ingested, the kidneys' concentrating ability, and extrarenal losses. Normal intake varies considerably and balances with urine output and other water losses (insensible losses, vomiting, diarrhea). The amount in a renal diet is determined by noting the dry body weight (that weight at which the patient has no signs of excess fluid) and prescribing fluid intake that permits excretion of solutes but does not result in symptomatic fluid overload.

Usual 24-hour allowance: Urine output guides fluid intake prescriptions. Often, 500 to 800 ml are added to the volume of urine voided in the previous 24 hours. This amount is in addition to the fluid found in solid food.

Fluids: Items that are liquid at room temperature: gelatin, ice cream, sherbet, popsicles, ice cubes and chips; as well as soup, syrup from canned fruit, liquid from vegetables; and beverages, liquid medicines, water taken with pills.

Cautions: Rapid changes in weight are usually indicative of rapid changes in fluid balance; 1000 ml of fluid equals 1 kg of body weight. Ice cubes and chips vary, so melt and measure a given volume of ice to determine intake.

Consider protein, sodium, and potassium levels in all liquids. Water, cranberry juice, Kool-Aid (not presweetened), and tea are low in unwanted substances.

Thirst causes discomfort so space liquids over 24 hours. This pattern also maintains GFR and urine output (the normal diurnal variation is lost). Offer cold liquids and provide materials for oral hygiene.

SODIUM

Function: Major extracellular fluid cation, important in acid-base balance, fluid balance, cell permeability, and muscle action.

Excess	Deficit
Hypernatremia	Hyponatremia
Edema	Dehydration
Hypertension	Hypotension
Congestive heart failure	

Desirable amount: A normal diet may have 3 to 10 g of sodium. The estimated daily requirement is 1 to 3 g. The amount in a renal diet is determined by considering the 24-hour losses in the urine as well as extrarenal losses (sweating, diarrhea) and blood pressure.

Usual 24-hour allowance: Sodium-restricted diets vary from 500 mg/day (strict), 1 g/day (moderate), 2 to 3 g/day (mild), to 4 g/day (no salt added).

1 g Na = 1000 mg Na
1 g NaCl = 400 mg Na
1 mEq Na = 23 mg Na

High sodium foods:

Table salt	Processed foods
Milk	Cured meat, fish, poultry
Meat	
Eggs	Pickled or brined foods
Carrots	Some canned soups,
Beets	vegetables
Spinach	Meat sauce, soy sauce
	Meat tenderizer
	Salad dressings

Other sources of sodium: Food additives such as baking soda, baking powder, salt, food preservatives; chewing tobacco or snuff; water softeners; and medicines such as cough syrup, pain relievers, laxatives, and antacids.

Cautions: Read all labels. Low sodium products are increasingly available. Watch for potassium levels in products such as salt substitute.

POTASSIUM

Function: Major intracellular fluid cation. Important in fluid balance, acid-base balance, neuromuscular activity, carbohydrate metabolism, and protein synthesis.

SODIUM CONTENT OF SELECTED MEDICATIONS

Drug	Manufacturer	Sodium content
Antacids		
Alka-Seltzer	Miles Lab	567 mg/tab
Soda mints	Lilly	87 mg/tab
Tums	Norcliff Thayer	≤2 mg/tab
Chooz	Plough	4 mEq/tab
Citrocarbonate	Upjohn	700 mg/4 g dose
Laxatives		
Fleet Phospho-Soda	Fleet	96.4 mEq/20 ml
Metamucil	Proctor & Gamble	1 mg/7 g (31 mg/7 g K+)
Metamucil Instant Mix (lemon-lime)	Proctor & Gamble	1 mg/packet (209 mg/packet K+)

Modified from Olin, BR, editor: Drug facts and comparisons, Philadelphia, 1990, JB Lippincott.

Excess	Deficit
Dangerous cardiac arrhythmias	Dangerous cardiac arrhythmias

Desirable amount: The estimated daily requirement normally is 1875 to 5625 mg; this may be increased with diarrhea. The amount in a renal diet depends on the kidneys' ability to excrete urine. The serum potassium level, the amount of potassium lost in the urine in 24 hours, and the level of acidosis are considered. If the urine output is equal to or greater than 800 ml/day, then usually potassium need not be restricted.

Usual 24-hour allowance: Renal diets restrict potassium to 1 mEq/kg ideal body weight per day or 40 to 60 mEq per day.

$$1 \text{ mEq K} = 39 \text{ mg K}$$
$$40 \text{ mEq K} = 1500 \text{ mg K}$$

High potassium foods:

Meat	Oranges	Potatoes
Whole grains	Bananas	Broccoli
Beans, nuts	Apricots	Spinach
Dried fruits	Melons	Peas
Fruit juices	Peaches	Tomatoes
	Avocados	

Other sources of potassium: Salt substitute, medicines such as antibiotics, beverages such as coffee and wine.

Cautions: Consider the amount of potassium in low-sodium foods.

PROTEINS

Function: Build, maintain, and repair body tissues.

Excess	Deficit
Uremic symptoms	Weight loss
High BUN	Low serum albumin levels

Desirable amount: Protein intake depends on the level of renal function, age, and physical activity. The recommended amount of protein per day for an adult man is 56 g, and for an adult woman it is 44 g. The usual American diet contains much more than this amount. The quality of protein, that is, high or low biologic value, is considered. In high biologic value (HBV) the nitrogen is in the form of the 8 essential amino acids and in roughly the proportions needed each day. These amino acids cannot be synthesized by the body and all must be present to build needed substances.

Usual 24-hour allowance: For patients with renal disorders, the amount of protein is determined by the level of renal function (creatinine clearance, 24-hour protein loss) and treatment modality (predialysis, hemodialysis, peritoneal dialysis, transplantation). In general, two thirds of the protein intake should be high biologic value and one third low biologic value.

Protein sources:

High biologic value (animal proteins)	Low biologic value (plant proteins)
Eggs	Grains (corn, wheat, rice)
Milk	
Meat	Legumes (dry beans, chick-peas, lentils, split peas, soybeans)
Fish	
Poultry	

Enteral nutrition products: Amin-Aid, Travasorb Renal
Parenteral nutrition products: Aminosyn RF, NephrAmine

Cautions: Adequate calories from carbohydrates and fats must also be available for the appropriate use of proteins. Protein needs increase with fever, infection, trauma. Consider the phosphorus in proteins.

CALORIES (CARBOHYDRATES, FATS)

Function: To meet body's need for energy and to attain or maintain ideal body weight. Fats are also important in maintaining skin integrity and forming complex lipid compounds. Major energy sources are carbohydrates (4 kcal/g) and fats (9 kcal/g). Protein provides 4 kcal/g. Using carbohydrates for fuel results in energy, water, and carbon dioxide. Fat, when oxidized completely, forms water and carbon dioxide. Otherwise excess acid metabolites such as ketoacids are formed.

Excess	Deficit
Weight gain	Weight loss
Satiety	Hunger

Desirable amount: The usual recommended caloric intake is 2300 to 3100 for men and 1600 to 2400 for women. Carbohydrate is required every day because stores (glycogen) are limited. Fat is required in the form of essential fatty acids; it is stored in adipose tissue. Amounts vary with age and activity. Carbohydrate and fat intake is increased in renal diets when protein is limited in order to provide adequate calories and prevent use of muscle protein for energy.

Usual 24-hour allowance: In renal diets, caloric intake generally is >35 kcal/kg of ideal body weight, with more from carbohydrate sources and less from fats. Amounts need to be increased with catabolic events such as fever and decreased when other sources of calories are part of the treatment (peritoneal dialysis).

Carbohydrate Sources:	Fat Sources:
Fruits	Butter, margarine, oil
Vegetables	Salad dressing
Cereals	Bacon, meat fat
Sugar	Cream
Hard candy, jelly	Egg yolk
beans	Olives, nuts, avocados
Jams, jellies	

Commercial high calorie/protein-free/low electrolyte products: Cal-Power, Hy-Cal

Cautions: Abnormal carbohydrate metabolism in renal disease causes carbohydrate intolerance with abnormal glucose utilization and altered insulin secretion and response. Abnormal lipid metabolism is associated with accelerated atherogenesis (increased production and decreased removal of low density lipids). Avoid fats high in saturated fats or cholesterol. Consider the amounts of protein, sodium, and potassium in high calorie foods. Diabetic patient must avoid concentrated sources of sweets.

VITAMIN AND MINERAL SUPPLEMENTS

Patients with renal disorders may become deficient in vitamins and minerals essential to good nutrition because of altered dietary intake or because of losses during dialysis.

Ascorbic acid (Vitamin C)

B complex vitamins (Thiamine, riboflavin, niacin, pantothenic acid, vitamin B12, folic acid, pyridoxine)

Calcium, phosphorus, and vitamin D: In addition to decreased intake, intestinal absorption of calcium is decreased, Vitamin D metabolism is abnormal, and parathyroid hormone secretion increases phosphorus levels. These interrelated factors contribute to alterations in blood clotting, bone metabolism, nerve conduction, muscle contraction, energy metabolism, and acid-base balance.

Calcium sources: Calcium carbonate (Os-Cal, Tums), calcium acetate (Phos-Lo), supplements given between meals.

Calcium supplements are based on calcium and phosphorus serum levels. Vitamin D is given with caution. If the levels of calcium and phosphorus are too high, that is, the product of the two concentrations ($[Ca] \times [P] > 70$), efforts are made to lower the phosphorus level because soft tissue calcification may occur. If renal osteodystrophy occurs, efforts are made to lower dietary phosphorus, too.

Phosphorus binding agents: Calcium acetate (Phos-Lo), aluminum hydroxide gel (Amphogel), aluminum carbonate (Basalgel), binding agents given with meals.

Vitamin D sources: Calciferol (Hytakerol), calcitriol (Rocaltrol)

Iron: Besides decreased intake, losses of this essential substance occur with repeated lab tests and hemodialysis. Extra iron is needed for patients receiving epoietin.

Iron sources: Ferrous sulfate, parenteral iron products.

Magnesium: Not usually a problem unless there is intake of magnesium-containing medicines such as laxatives and antacids.

Cautions: Fat-soluble vitamins are not usually needed. A toxic amount of vitamin A can be ingested if not excluded from the multiple vitamin preparation ordered for the patient.

• • •

Tables A-1, A-2, and A-3 include a summary of dietary alterations considered for acute renal failure, chronic renal failure, nephrotic syndrome, renal calculi, diabetic nephropathy, hemodialysis, peritoneal dialysis, and after renal transplantation. This information is included for comparison purposes only and should not be used for individual patient decisions.

Table A-1

COMPARISON OF GENERAL DIET MODIFICATIONS FOR ACUTE AND CHRONIC RENAL FAILURE

Nutrients	Acute Renal Failure	Chronic Renal Failure
Fluids	Urine volume plus 500 ml/day	Balanced with output to avoid edema
Sodium	40-90 mEq/day, depends on BP	60-90 mEq/day, depends on BP
Potassium	≤60 mEq/day with hyperkalemia	40-70 mEq/day or 1 mEq per g protein
Protein	0.4-0.6 g/kg/day	0.4-0.6 g/kg/day plus 24-h protein loss
	1-1.5 g/kg/day if on dialysis (70% HBV)	(75% HBV)
Calories (CHO, fat)	Sufficient to maintain weight	>35 kcal/kg/day
		Sufficient to attain or maintain ideal body weight; nonprotein kcal i.e., 50% CHO, remaining from fat
Vitamins	B complex, C, folate, not A	B complex, C, folate, not A
Minerals Ca	1400-1600 mg/day	1400-1600 mg/d
P	4-10 mg/kg/day	8-17 mg/kg/d

Compiled from references 17, 20, 29.
Note: *HBV*, high biologic value; *CHO*, carbohydrates

Table A-2

GENERAL DIET MODIFICATIONS FOR NEPHROTIC SYNDROME, DIABETIC NEPHROPATHY, RENAL CALCULI

Nutrients	Modifications(s)
Nephrotic syndrome	
Fluids	Depends on renal function
Sodium	60-90 mEq/day, depending on edema
Potassium	No restriction, usually
Protein	0.8-1 g/kg/day, more if malnourished, plus 24-h protein loss
Calories	Attain or maintain ideal body weight (edema-free); mostly complex CHO; limit fats to 30% of calories, limit cholesterol
Vitamins/Minerals	As needed
Diabetic nephropathy	
Fluids	Depends on renal function
Sodium	Depends on edema, blood pressure
Potassium	No restriction, usually
Protein	About 10% of calories; 0.6 g/kg/day (HBV), plus 24-h protein loss
Calories	35 kcal/kg/ideal body weight, CHO: 60%, complex forms, simple forms used with care and spread to avoid peaks and valleys in glycemic control; (renal diet needs are priority)
	Fat: about 30% of calories, <10% saturated fat
Vitamins/Minerals	As needed
Renal Calculi	
Fluids	250-300 ml/h while awake and once during night; 50% as water
Sodium	Restricted moderately with hypercalciuria; with thiazide diuretics 90 mEq/day
Purines	Avoid excessive amounts of meat, fish, poultry, especially organ meats; dried beans, lentils, bran; avoid fat and alcohol
Oxalate	Less than 50 mg/day; avoid tea, cocoa, beans, nuts, selected fruits and vegetables
Vitamins/Minerals	Restricted with calcium and oxalate stones
	Low calcium diet: 400-600 mg/day
	Moderate calcium diet: 800 mg/day

Compiled from references 17, 20, 29.
Note: CHO, carbohydrates; HBV, high biologic value.

Table A-3

A COMPARISON OF DIET MODIFICATIONS FOR SELECTED TREATMENT MODALITIES IN CHRONIC RENAL FAILURE

Nutrients	Hemodialysis	Peritoneal Dialysis	Renal Transplantation
Fluids	Urine volume plus 500 ml	Generally not restricted	Not restricted
Sodium	500-3000 mg/day	2000-3000 mg/day as tolerated, i.e., weight, BP	Usually not restricted
Potassium	2000-3000 mg/day, depends on K^+ in dialysate	3000-3500 mg/day, unless high serum K^+, more if peritonitis	Not restricted
Protein	1.2-1.4 g/kg/day 50% HBV	1.2-1.5 g/kg/day More with peritonitis	1.2-1.5 g/kg/day
Calories	To maintain or attain ideal weight $\geq$35 kcal/kg/day	35-42 kcal/kg/day minus kcal from dialysate	Control to avoid excessive weight gain
CHO	50% of kcal		50% of kcal
Fat	Rest of nonprotein kcal	35% of kcal	30-35% of kcal Limit cholesterol
Vitamins	Water soluble only, folate, D3, if needed	Water soluble only, folate, D3, if needed	Multiple vitamins
Minerals	**Supplement or restrict based on body levels**		
Calcium	1200-1800 mg/day	1000-1400 mg/day	1200 mg/day
Phosphorus	600-1200 mg/day	800-1200 mg/day	1200 mg/day
Iron	As needed	As needed	

Compiled from references 17, 20, 29.
Note: HBV, high biologic value; CHO, carbohydrates

References

1. Bennett WM: *Drugs and renal disease*, ed 2, New York, 1986, Churchill-Livingstone.
1a. Brundage DJ: *Nursing management of renal problems*, ed 2, St. Louis, 1980, Mosby–Year Book.
2. Canobbio MM: *Cardiovascular disorders*, St. Louis, 1990, Mosby–Year Book.
3. Catto GRD, editor: *New clinical applications in nephrology: Transplantation*, Dordrecht, 1989, Kluwer Academic Publishers.
4. Centers for Disease Control: Extrapulmonary tuberculosis cases by site, states, 1989. Personal communication, 1991.
5. Cunha BA, Friedman PE: Antibiotic dosing in patients with renal insufficiency or receiving dialysis, *Heart Lung* 17(6):612-616, 1988.
6. deKernion JB, Paulson DF: *Genitourinary cancer management*, Philadelphia, 1987, Lea & Febiger.
7. Earle DA, Levin ML, Quintanilla AP, editors: *Manual of clinical nephrology*, Philadelphia, 1982, WB Saunders.
8. Eble JN, editor: *Tumors and tumor-like conditions of the kidneys and ureters*, New York, 1990, Churchill Livingstone.
9. Fowler JE Jr.: *Manual of urologic surgery*, Boston, 1990, Little, Brown.
10. Fowler JE Jr., Lee M, Caldamone AA: *Urinary tract infection and inflammation*, Chicago, 1989, Mosby–Year Book.
11. Gillenwater JJ, Grayhack JT, Howards SS, and Duckett JW, editors: *Adult and pediatric urology*, vol 1, St. Louis, 1991, Mosby–Year Book.
12. Johnson DL: Nephrotic syndrome: a nursing care plan based on current pathophysiologic concepts, *Heart Lung* 18(1):85-92, 1989.
12a. Karb VB, Queener SF, Freeman JB: *Handbook of drugs for nursing practice*, St. Louis, 1989, Mosby–Year Book.
13. Kissane JM, editor: *Anderson's pathology*, ed 8, St. Louis, 1985, Mosby–Year Book.
14. Klahr S, editor: *The kidney and body fluids in health and disease*, New York, 1983, Plenum Medical Books.
15. Lewis SM, Collier IC: *Medical-surgical nursing: assessment and management of clinical problems*, ed 2, St. Louis, 1987, Mosby–Year Book.
16. McCance KL, Huether SE: *Pathophysiology: the biologic basis for disease in adults and children*, St. Louis, 1990, Mosby–Year Book.
17. Mitch WE, Klahr S, editors: *Nutrition and the kidney*, Boston, 1988, Little, Brown.
18. Mourad LA: *Orthopedic disorders*, St. Louis, 1991, Mosby–Year Book.
19. Muehrcke RC: *Acute renal failure*, St. Louis, 1969, Mosby–Year Book.
20. Pemberton CM, Moxness KE, German MJ, et al: *Mayo Clinic diet manual: a handbook of dietary practices*, ed 6, Toronto, 1988, BC Decker.
21. Preuss HG, editor: *Management of common problems in renal disease*, New York, 1988, Macmillan.
22. Seeley RR, Stephens TD, and Tate P: *Anatomy and physiology*, St. Louis, 1989, Mosby–Year Book.
23. Seidel HM, Ball JW, Dains JE, and Benedict GW: *Mosby's guide to physical examination*, ed 2, St. Louis, 1991, Mosby–Year Book.
24. Sweny P, Farrington K, and Moorhead JF: *The kidney and its disorders*, Oxford, 1989, Blackwell Scientific Publications.
25. Tanagho EA, McAinich JW: *Smith's general urology*, ed 12, Norwalk, Conn, 1988, Appleton & Lange.
26. Thelan LA, Davie JK, and Urden LD: *Textbook of critical care nursing*, St. Louis, 1990, Mosby–Year Book.
26a. Thibodeau GA: *Anatomy and physiology*, St. Louis, 1987, Mosby–Year Book.
27. Thompson JM, McFarland GK, Hirsch JE, Tucker SM, and Bowers AC: *Mosby's manual of clinical nursing*, ed 2, St. Louis, 1989, Mosby–Year Book.
28. United States Renal Data System: *The second annual report of the United States Renal Data System, 1990*, prepared in cooperation with the Urban Institute, Washington, DC, and University of Michigan, Ann Arbor.
29. Zeman FJ: *Clinical nutrition and dietetics*, ed 2, New York, 1991, Macmillan.

Index